What people ar

No Matter What ... I *Still* Win

Lia Young vividly recounts her journey from a healthy woman with a happy young family to being suddenly struck with a terminal lung disease that ultimately causes her to need a double lung transplant. She chronicles the trials and tribulations of navigating through the health care system to get her lung disease correctly diagnosed and to be placed on a waitlist for double lung transplants. This is an extraordinary real-life story: a story of love, loss, and resilience; of family, friendship, and faith. It is an inspiring story for people of all walks of life, and especially for people who need organ transplants and those who care for them.

Si Pham, MD, Mayo Clinic, Jacksonville, Florida

I would recommend this story to anyone who is going through health issues, facing impossible odds, insecurity and fear of the future, or just wondering what God is up to in their life. Everyone needs to learn that with Jesus, no matter what, we still win!

Jim Markle, DEdMin, Director of Administration for Christian Community Action

Very seldom are there books with as much power and as much transparency as this book. Robert and Lia have truly bared their lives and their souls to the reader. This compelling page turner is one that will inspire you, cause you to do some serious self-evaluation, and empower you to make it through every trial you face. It proves that you can finish what you start. Despite the most challenging difficulties, they made sure they completed this book. I recommend it not just once but as your go-to when you face the ups and downs of life. There is Hope. There is Victory. We Still Win!

Sonjia B. Dickerson, Pastor
of Dayspring Family Church,
Irving, Texas

This book is really inspiring, encouraging, and uplifting. I remember everything we went through, and it is amazing that we made it through. You (Lia) and Daddy worked so hard on this book. Even if I weren't your (Lia's) daughter, I would read it.

Raelyn Young, Lia's daughter,
age 10

I boarded a plane for a missionary trip to Africa in tears fearing I would never see my friend Lia again. I prayed and pleaded that somehow in the eleventh hour Lia would make it through. Hope beyond all hope and probability! You can imagine my elation when the news reached me across the world that Lia was miraculously breathing again! I was blessed with a front row seat to see Lia's faith beckon her from the shallow end of the life's pool into the unpredictable depths of overflowing grace and strength. With every valid excuse to complain, become a victim and give up, Lia learned how to truly catch her breath. Every Sunday at church there she was with her oxygen tank praising God, loving people, and moving past her pain. This book is the friend you've prayed for to challenge you and whisper truth in the middle of your dark night. As Lia's story touches your heart, you'll feel like someone's forged a path before you, leaving markers of hope along the way. She is a champion, and her story will embolden you to rise up through your own challenges to win again!

Kris White, Sr. Pastor of
The Bridge Church, Denton, Texas

Real, raw, and riveting. These words flood my mind about Lia's compelling story. It's been my honor to journey through this adventure with Robert and Lia as their pastor. We have laughed and cried. Rejoiced and mourned. Through it all, together we have overcome. I have witnessed firsthand how Lia's faith and tenacity have transformed her into the hero she is today. As you delve into the roller coaster ride of Lia's story, you will encounter a fierce breed of hope. That hope will become an anchor for your own soul to strengthen and inspire you in your storm. Then will you realize—you can still win too!

Duane White, Sr. Pastor of
The Bridge Church, Denton,
Texas

NO MATTER WHAT...
I *Still* WIN

A STORY OF LUNGS, LOSS AND LOVE

LIA YOUNG
LiaYoung.com

Levo Press

NO MATTER WHAT … I *STILL* WIN
Published by Levo Press
539 W. Commerce
Ste. 707
Dallas, TX 75208

LevoPress.com

info@levopress.com

©2019 by Lia Young

All rights reserved. Except for brief excerpts for review purposes, no part of this book may be reproduced or used in any form without written permission from the publisher.

All Scripture quotations, unless otherwise noted, are taken from the *Holy Bible, New International Version®. NIV®.* Copyright ©1973, 1984, 2011 by Biblica, Inc™. Used by permission of Zondervan. All rights reserved. Scripture quotations marked "ESV" are taken from *The Holy Bible, English Standard Version®* (ESV®), copyright ©2000; 2001 by Crossway, a division of Good News Publishers. Used by permission. All rights reserved.

Cover Design: Air Designs
Author Photo: Allyson Rhodes

ISBN 978-1-7907-2905-0

Printed in the United States of America
First Edition 2019

1 2 3 4 5 6 7 8 9 10

To my Love, Robert. You're the best part.

Acknowledgments

Over the past eight years, my family and I have been the recipients of tremendous support and prayers. There are hundreds, if not thousands, of people, businesses, churches, and foundations whom I have thanked for keeping us prayed up, fed, loved, and financially stable through my health challenges. Writing a book was something that I always wanted to do, even before my first sign of "pneumonia," but I didn't know what it should or would be about. God has provided a beautiful story for me to tell, and He continues to allow me to experience its unfolding every day. I deeply appreciate the following people who helped me get this book from my head to your shelf or digital device ...

Most importantly, I want to thank God that I'm alive to tell this story. There have been countless moments when my life could easily have become a memory, but I am still here, and I'm thankful that He has kept me through it all.

My husband, Robert, told me time and time again to write this book. "Babe, you gotta tell your story," he'd say, "You never know who you could inspire ... who's gonna look at you overcoming and get through their own struggles because of you." Robert saved my life and made me a walking miracle. He never gave up on me. He encouraged me. Supported me. Left me alone so I could write, and genuinely showed interest in what I was thinking, dreaming, and writing. Writing this book provided many opportunities for the two of us to share deeply intimate conversations that I will forever cherish.

Jimmy and Sharron Jackson with Levo Press … Sharron, thank you for being excited about my story and for being a constant encourager to put my pen to paper. Thank you for being a voice of reason and making sure I was transparent enough to paint the picture for the reader without being offensive. Thank you for making connections between my life experiences and God's Word, which helped me discover some things about myself. Jimmy, thank you for supporting this book, for your marketing and promotional efforts, and for being even more excited about the possibilities and impact this book will have than I am. (Who knew that was possible?) I am so excited about the lives this story will touch.

Allyson Rhodes at Air Designs, thank you for taking my story and ideas and turning them into tangible cover art. I continue to be amazed by your creativity and appreciate your expertise. To Ryan Honeywell, thank you for lending your creative genius to this project. How you were able to portray my story in a minute and a half video blows my mind! But you did, and you did it well.

Darryl Tomlinson, Alex Pugh, Todd Mohair, Shon Hughes, Tamara Russell, and Talibah Anderson … Thank you for filling in the blanks in my story when Robert could not. I'm so thankful that he confided in you and that you were able to share his perspective with me.

Contents

Prologue   13

1. You Had Me at "Whataburger"   17
2. Negroes Can't Swim   23
3. We'll Just Call It "Pneumonia"   27
4. We Is Pregnant Now!   37
5. "You Don't Look So Good"   41
6. I'm Alive, But What Happened?   48
7. What You Talkin' 'Bout Doc?   55
8. Going, Going. Back, Back. To Texas, Texas.   61
9. Can't Win for Losing   66
10. Lookin' For Lungs   73
11. Houston … I Have a Problem   82
12. Hitting the Wall Face First   87
13. Shouting at My Mountain   96
14. I'm Leaving on a Jet Plane   114
15. Blessed and Highly Favored   123
16. Living Our Best Life   136
17. … And Now This?   140

Epilogue   149
Frequently Asked Questions   151
Medical Terms Glossary   162

Prologue

"YOU NEED TO WRITE A BOOK."

This is the statement I've heard over and over from the moment I realized I was alive with new pre-owned lungs until now. My husband, Robert, was my number one encourager in writing this book and making sure I followed through. We frequently shared our story with friends, strangers, and others going through medical challenges. Over and over, people confirmed that our story was something we must share. It helped equip others to face their own situations with wisdom and courage. It was inspiring. Riveting. Miraculous. So, in July 2018, I finally picked up my pen. It was time to share our story and make this journey known to the masses.

I had already given the book the working title *I Still Win*. It was not our goal to get rich off royalties but to inspire others to strengthen their faith, advocate for themselves and those they love, and never give up. (But, let's be serious, a bestseller or movie deal wouldn't be a bad thing!) Robert and I met with our friends, Sharron and Jimmy, who became our editorial and marketing team. And I began writing.

In early September, I finished writing my perspective of everything that happened from the first scary cough to our life after my double lung transplant. It was therapeutic for me to reminisce and review each step of the way. As I wrote, Robert and I talked about what he remembered and experienced during that part of the story. I completed my contribution a little ahead of schedule, submitted it for editing, and started jotting down Robert's perspective. We decided to structure the book so that the reader could read what I was experiencing and thinking but could also see what Robert was going through at that time. The day after I submitted my story to Sharron for editing, Robert and I spent time discussing his thoughts. He didn't want to forget anything important that could be included in the book.

We snuck away from the house for coffee that night. When we returned, "Back Down Memory Lane" by Minnie Riperton was on the radio. We sat in the driveway, and Robert began to tell me how the song came on one night after he had returned from seeing me at the hospital. The doctors had just told him it was unlikely I would make it through the night. It was his duty to come home and tell the family—our children— that Mommy might not make it. He told me how the song prompted him to think of all the times we had shared, the memories we'd made, and the things I was going to miss. He said he had sat in the car sobbing and had to get himself together just to go in the house. I'm so glad Robert shared this with me. I had always wondered how he held up while I was sick. I wondered if he ever broke down … if that gorgeous smile ever disappeared. I made a mental note of his story, and we went into the house. Little did I know that over the next two days, I would face the most unexpected and intense storm of them all.

———————————

Here I am, and here is my story. It's not the story I thought it would be, and it's not the story I would have chosen. But I pray it will encourage you to live your own story to its fullest. I pray that by its end you, too, will join me in declaring over your own life that No Matter What ... I *Still* Win!

ONE

You Had Me At "Whataburger"

OUR STORY BEGINS IN 1997. I was an 18-year-old country girl from Palestine, Texas who had made it to the "big city" of Denton to study nursing at Texas Woman's University (TWU). Robert was a 23-year-old native of Denton, a "Denton-ite." My orientation leaders had warned us about Denton-ites. Supposedly, they knew all the nooks and crannies in Denton and took innocent college girls there to do obscene things with them.

It was late in the afternoon one Saturday when my friends and I realized we had a few minutes left before the Student Union closed, and we hadn't eaten. We stopped playing beauty shop and watching movies and headed out of the dorm to get some grub. We looked casual, very casual. You might even say we looked "tore up from the floor up." After grabbing our food, we headed back to the dorm along Bell Avenue, the main street running through campus. About halfway down the street, a green Mitsubishi Eclipse with tinted windows and three black faces peering out from inside pulled in front of us. They let down the window and two of my friends bolted car side. My best friend Tamara and I stayed on the sidewalk, remembering the warning our well-meaning university staff had given us just months before. Then a voice from the passenger side yelled out, "Hey, Blackie … come over here! Ain't nobody gonna rape you." I assumed he was talking to me because my bestie is light-skinned. I worked my neck, looked at Tamara, and said, "Oh no, he didn't … lookin' like the Pillsbury Doughboy."

We slowly approached the passenger side and met "Shon." After talking for a few minutes, we traded numbers. Our plan was to go to the movies as a group the next weekend. On Saturday, we all met up, traveled to Dallas, and went to the movies. On the ride down, "Shon" informed me that his name was actually Robert and that he had a one-year-old daughter named Jasmine. I was like "whatever" because I really wasn't interested in him anyway. Besides, at 18, I didn't want to deal with baby mama drama or motherhood. To be honest, I simply saw this night out as an opportunity for me—a broke college student—to get some free entertainment.

Robert and I had a lot of fun together that night, and soon, a simple opportunity for a free movie turned into something so much more. Robert was funny and entertaining. Most importantly, he could cook. From the first time he handed me his debit card at

Whataburger and told me to order anything I wanted (even a milkshake with my combo!), I knew he was the one. I had fallen in love.

We dated for seven years and made a lot of memories together. Long before we had even thought of marriage, many of our friends told us we had similar personalities and were perfect for each other. At our base, we were and, until Robert's passing, continued to be true friends. Robert was the best friend anyone could have. He was Mr. Friendly everywhere he went and truly never met a stranger. Robert was the guy in Wal-Mart hugging, waving, and talking to everybody. When I'd ask him, "Who was that?" he'd reply, "I don't know."

Robert was also much more forgiving and generous than I. He always offered his time and talents to his friends. Earlier in our relationship I often told him he needed to learn to say "no" and start thinking about the impact his generosity towards others might have on his own life. I'd ask him, "Why do you have to be the one that everybody in the family calls?" And, "So, you said *we* would host the barbecue?" In even the most ordinary, everyday things, Robert always went that extra step to make it the very best it could be, even when something less would have sufficed. For example, he could never just make a basic macaroni and cheese. He had to add four different cheeses, thick-cut applewood smoked bacon, and a breadcrumb topping. Now, I never complained, and I gladly ate it, but I would have been content with the basic mac 'n' cheese from the blue box.

If you did Robert wrong, he didn't cut you off. Instead, he put you in rotation. He gave people a lot more opportunities to be his friend than I would have. In fact, I'm somewhat of the opposite in the friend department. Over the years of being around and observing Robert, I learned to be more outgoing. I am now conscious of my body posture and facial expressions and learned early on that there is a difference between being direct and being downright rude. My tone of voice is a work in progress. I like to be well informed, organized, and on time. Robert always stored things in his head and never showed when he was stressed. Timeliness was always a sensitive subject between us. One of the first things his friends told me on our first group date was that he was never on time.

Robert and I experienced a lot of happy moments together like traveling, new cars, my first apartment, hanging with friends, and becoming adults. With each hill, there were also valleys. We experienced many difficult situations and turbulent times throughout the early years of our relationship: nursing school, bad bosses, sick family members, and the passing of loved ones. Then there were Robert's marriage, divorce, and two additional children—Telia and Robert Jr. Those five rollercoaster years of hell are another story for another book. Perhaps I'll title it *No Matter What … I Still Win: The Original Story.*

During those early years, we prayed a lot and attended church often. As our faith in God grew stronger through each trial, our relationship with each other also grew closer and stronger. We weren't Bible scholars, but we knew God and we knew He was good. We always trusted Him to help a brotha' or a sista' out, and over and over, that's exactly what He did.

We purchased our first home in 2004 soon after our engagement and got married in 2005. Our first child together, Raelyn (aka Rae Rae), was born in 2009. Robert and I knew our roles in our relationship. He worked, planned fun events and travel, transported the kids to and from school, managed all car care, and coordinated the kids' sports activities.

Most importantly to me, and integral to the operations of our home, Robert did the grocery shopping and cooking. He was an incredible cook, always found deals, and bought in bulk. Kroger was his thinking ground, and he made daily trips to clear his head and peruse the clearance aisle. Shortly after we moved into our home, I realized he was the chef and I was the sous chef. He would peer over my shoulder as I cooked and instruct me to sauté a little longer or add this or that. I finally gave him the reins and resolved to chop vegetables, organize the pantry, and do the dishes.

Shortly before we got married, Robert left corporate America and opened his own copier consulting business, so he could work from home and have a more flexible schedule for his kids. He also played the good cop when we bought a car. I kept us organized, made all the service calls, worked, coordinated our health benefits, did laundry, made sure the kids were registered for school and had all their supplies, and made certain we paid the bills on time. I played the bad cop when we bought a car. I also provided emotional support to the kids, especially to Raelyn. Even when she was very young, she always needed that extra Mom talk—the talk-her-off-the-edge and take-a-deep-breath-to-calm-down talk. Rae Rae has always needed to know that everything is going to be okay, even when she can't find her purple sock or her lucky soccer headband.

From the start, Robert and I just fit. We were a well-oiled machine, the perfect team. We were best friends.

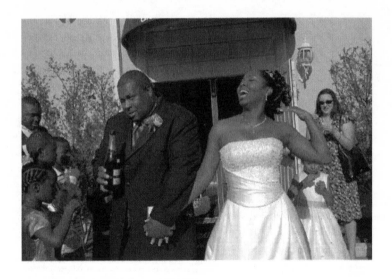

TWO

Negroes Can't Swim

IN 2011, WE DECIDED TO SELL our first home. We were going to build a house big enough to accommodate all the kids with a few bells and whistles. We also knew we wanted at least one more child, so getting a bigger home was important. Our house sold so fast we didn't have time to secure a place to live during the time between the sale of the old house and the completion of the new one. At that time, it was nearly impossible to find a short-term or month-to-month lease anywhere. So, we ended up in a single-wide trailer. It was what Robert had always wanted (really!). This was our running joke. He would tell me stories about visiting his uncle's trailer back in the day. The a/c blew freezing, cold air from floor vents, and to Robert's childhood self, trailer living was a dream. He always knew how to sell me on something. "They're just like homes," he would tell me, "just mobile!"

It was hilarious seeing my BMW 750Li sitting in the driveway of a mobile home. But, it was super cheap, had freezing, cold air blowing out of the floor vents just as Robert remembered, provided just enough room for our family, and was minutes from where our new home was being built. It was late June, and it was hot. We packed up our home and moved most of our belongings to storage and the absolute necessities to the trailer. We had so much going on we decided to cancel our vacation to Los Angeles and go instead on an in-state trip to Sea World in San Antonio.

After settling into the trailer life, we headed to San Antonio in July. We met up with another family there and had a blast together. All the kids and our nephew Jamaras, who has been our plus-one for much of his life, came along. Sea World had recently opened a waterpark section, and I had never been to a waterpark in my life. I figured I'd be the cool Mom and ride the waterslide with the kids. We climbed an endless metal staircase until we were so high Robert and Rae Rae looked like tiny ants where they stood watching us from below. Robert Jr. and Jamaras went first. Next, I approached the slide cautiously. Carefully following the lifeguard's instructions, I laid down on my back and crossed my arms over my chest. The water began rushing all around me, and away I went, swirling and twirling down that gigantic, plastic tube for what seemed like ten minutes until I reached what felt like a hill in the tube. "I must be near the end of this terrible decision," I thought. Suddenly, the hill propelled me into the air. I closed my eyes, screamed, and continued that scream until I felt water splash around me and eventually over my head. I remember trying to find my bearings and working to get my feet under me. Finally, I stood up, flung my hair out of my face, and began wiping the water out of my eyes. My mouth was so full of water I started spitting it out and began to cough. I made it to the walkway where Jamaras and Robert Jr. stood waiting for me, a look of shock on their faces. I continued to cough and spew out water. At last I caught my breath and half joked, "Whew! I'm probably gonna catch pneumonia with all that water I just aspirated!" A few hours later we left Sea World and have never been back.

We returned home and began preparing for the kids to start school. The builder had broken ground on our second home. We had prayed over the lot and were busy picking out tile, flooring, and carpet. I was planning to start refereeing another season of basketball in the fall, but over the next few weeks, I noticed it was becoming more difficult to take the stairs at work. My joints were really sore, but I just chalked it up to getting older and not working out in a while. I was a whopping thirty-three at the time. I kept doing my regular day-to-day tasks, using Motrin, Bengay, Aspercream, and whatever else I could find to ease the joint pain.

Then one morning I woke up with more soreness in my joints than ever before. I pulled back the sheets, and both my legs were swollen with pitting edema. (Pitting edema is when you put your finger on your leg, remove it, and the imprint stays.) My legs were so big they didn't look like they belonged on my body. The skin on my knees and elbows were black and ashen, and there were dead flakes I could peel off. My fingers were swollen to the size of hot links. I thought to myself, "This is not normal." When I tried to stand up, one of my legs gave out. Thankfully, I caught myself with the help of the bed and called out to Robert. I didn't know what was going on, but I knew something was definitely wrong.

THREE

We'll Just Call It "Pneumonía"

BEING A NURSE, I DIDN'T PANIC. I assessed the situation and problem solved. Maybe my body had swelled up like a balloon because I was experiencing an allergic reaction to something, or maybe I had eaten an excessive amount of salt. So, I hobbled to our medicine cabinet and found Motrin, Benadryl, and a thermometer. I wasn't running a temp, and I wasn't in pain, but I figured somewhere I was inflamed, so I took 600mg of Motrin. Then I took 50mg of Benadryl to help reverse the effect of any allergen I might be reacting to. Why I didn't go to the emergency room that very second, I don't know. Maybe they could have run some blood tests to figure out what was happening, which could have prevented everything we went through in 2016. That instant decision not to go get immediate help is one that would always make me wonder.

Several hours later I awoke from my Benadryl-induced slumber. All the swelling was gone, my skin was back to normal, and I could walk without a problem. That incident never happened again, but it prompted me to call my primary care provider first thing Monday morning and schedule an appointment.

The appointment was set for a few days later. I met with my primary care doctor and gave her the story of what had happened over the weekend. No family history of anything autoimmune. No arthritis. No blood disorders. No bone injuries, breaks, or surgeries. One uneventful pregnancy, which resulted in a normal, healthy baby. No meds other than birth control and occasional Tylenol or Motrin for headaches and Benadryl for allergies. She did a full head-to-toe assessment and informed me that I looked great. Everything sounded good, except for a few crackles she heard in the base of one of my lungs.

"Do you have a respiratory history?" she asked.

"No," I answered quickly, "not even asthma, but I do think I aspirated some water at Sea World about a month ago."

She told me that there was definitely something in that lung and ordered an x-ray. She told me to keep doing what I was doing and let her know if I experienced any symptoms like the previous weekend again. I took the x-ray order to the hospital across the street, and they whisked me to the back. I took off my shirt, conscious to make sure everything was tucked in and covered. The tech took the x-ray, both AP (front-to-back image) and LAT (side-to-side image), and I was on my way. Within an hour, my doctor called me and said that a small pocket of fluid was noted in the lower lobe of one of my lungs. It wasn't big but could get worse, so she ordered breathing treatments and antibiotics. I proceeded to take my medications, but after a week with no improvement, I went back to my doctor. She ordered another x-ray. I went back to the hospital, had the x-ray done, and waited on the results.

It turned out that the pocket of fluid in the first lung was now bigger, and there was something brewing in the second lung. She decided to send me to a pulmonologist and called in prescriptions for a new antibiotic, steroids, and more albuterol for breathing treatments. Handing me a piece of paper with about five doctors' names listed on it, she pointed to the name circled in red. "I would choose this one," she said. "He's local, and I hear he's really nice." So, I called the pulmonologist she recommended and scheduled an appointment for the next week. His office said this would give him time to get my records and review them. A week later I went to the pulmonologist's office hopeful he would be able to tell what was wrong with me. I told him all about the incident that happened that Saturday morning and the course of action taken so far. He was very kind. He listened to my chest, had me do several breathing tests, and ordered a CT scan. The images from the CT scan revealed I had fluid pockets in both lungs. The pulmonologist prescribed more antibiotics and steroids and instructed me to follow up with him in a week if things did not improve.

Over the next week, nothing really changed. I was still having some shortness of breath, and everyday tasks left me feeling mildly fatigued. But I never had a fever, my joints were not as sore as they had been, and the boost of steroids made me feel like Wonder Woman (at least some of the time). I went back to the pulmonologist, and he proposed I get a bronchoscopy done. A bronchoscopy is when a doctor sticks a tube down the throat into the lungs, looks around, and takes a sample from the lining of the lungs. Doctors also use the procedure to wash the lungs out, take a sample of that fluid, test it, and determine what's wrong. The pulmonologist decided he would do the bronchoscopy within the next couple days and told me the scheduler for the hospital would get back with me with the exact date and time. I remember sitting on the steps of our temporary trailer home calling the hospital where I worked as Assistant Director of Nursing to let them know I would need to be off the next day for my procedure.

I went home, did a Google search for "bronchoscopy," and looked at videos I probably shouldn't have to prepare myself for the next day. On the morning of the procedure, Robert and I headed to the hospital. Someone on the medical team had told us it would be a 30-minute procedure, and the prep would take longer than the actual procedure. My nurse in the pre-op area was our wedding coordinator at the venue where we got married. As she readied me for the procedure, we reminisced about our wedding and all the life events that had happened since that day.

The anesthesiologist entered the room when I was all prepped. I signed my consent forms, and he fed some happy juice through my IV. Before the nurse rolled me out of the room, I was already sleepy. Next, I remember my pulmonologist telling me to count down from ten to one. I think I made it to eight.

Robert sat in the waiting room and watched as people who had come in after us left with their loved ones. Time passed. Too much time. And Robert began to wonder what was wrong. Then my doctor appeared at the door. Robert said later that the doctor had a look of shock on his face. He pulled Robert into a small conference room near the entrance of the day surgery area and asked, "Did Lia ever cough up blood?"

"No," Robert replied.

"I'm asking this because once we got to her vocal cords, she started hemorrhaging blood. Has she ever had any problems with anesthesia?"

"No," Robert again replied.

Then my doctor assured Robert everything would be okay and went back into the surgery area.

About an hour later, I woke up in the post-op area gasping for air, somewhat delusional, and crying. I didn't know what had happened. I just didn't feel right. The nurses in their blue bonnets and surgical scrubs came to my bedside to comfort me. I remember one of them saying, "Girl! You scared us."

And I thought to myself, "Y'all are scaring me right now."

Then the nurse began telling me what happened in the operating room. She explained that they had aborted the procedure because I was hemorrhaging so much. She also told me I would have to stay in the hospital at least a day for monitoring. I requested to see

31

Robert, and he hustled back to me. I immediately saw a look of fear on his face. After three days in the hospital, I was discharged home.

My doctors were unable to determine what was in my lungs, so they continued treating it as pneumonia. Soon after we arrived home, I noticed swelling in my chest above my breasts, and my neck was big and swollen like that of an NFL offensive lineman. My nose was congested, and when I talked, I sounded like a chipmunk. It was as though my throat was closing, and I couldn't get air through. When I pressed on my chest, it crackled like rice cereal. In the medical community, we call this crepitus. I had a follow-up appointment with my pulmonologist the next day and planned to bring up the changes I had noticed. At that appointment, he told me my condition was very concerning, especially the change in my voice. He informed me that I probably had air trapped in my chest cavity that was pushing on my trachea, causing tracheal deviation. I was immediately admitted to the hospital, so they could rule out a pneumothorax (collapsed lung) or pulmonary embolism (a blood clot in the lungs). The hospital staff completed several x-rays and CT scans on me, which revealed flurries throughout my lungs and fluid pockets at the bases. They gave me large doses of antibiotics and steroids. There was even talk about placing a chest tube in my left side to relieve fluid built up around my lung. Thankfully, it was not enough fluid to warrant a chest tube. They ruled out a pneumothorax or pulmonary embolism, but I still stayed in the hospital for over a week.

While I was in the hospital, the infectious disease doctors visited to get my medical history in hopes that they could determine what was wrong. They asked me so many questions I started to question myself. *Was I in a monogamous relationship? Did I ever have a pet bird? Had I researched what chemicals were used in the pools at Sea World?* I was finally discharged home with a specific drug regimen, which included steroids, antibiotics, breathing treatments, and oxygen. It was the first time I had to use portable oxygen. The oxygen vendor brought liquid oxygen to the trailer. It was quite the sight, like a scene straight from *Mork & Mindy*! The tank was about four feet tall and eighteen inches in diameter. It had these huge railings around the top that made it look like a keg. I had a 25-foot nasal cannula— tubing connecting the oxygen tank to my nostrils— which allowed me to walk from one end of the trailer to the other. I think my settings were at two or four liters per minute at that time. I also had a portable cylinder of liquid oxygen that I filled and took with me when I ran errands. However, it was only good for about two hours. I was a little intimidated the first couple times I filled up the portable oxygen. Liquid oxygen can get very cold, and it makes a distinct sound like air brakes when you put it into a portable tank. My doctor also told me to watch my salt and sugar intake during this time because the steroids could make me gain weight.

I followed up with my pulmonologist about every three weeks. In the meantime, I sought second opinions. I went to a pulmonologist in Dallas, and though he also didn't know what I had, he agreed with my current course of treatment. I also saw an immunologist, thinking maybe I had some weird autoimmune disease or allergy. She found nothing. Next, I saw a rheumatologist, thinking maybe my issues were caused by some type of arthritis or lupus. He also had no answers.

My status was unchanged. My oxygen saturation (O2 sats) with activity remained lower than desired but recovered fairly quickly with rest. I still coughed occasionally, and the flurries that had appeared on my chest x-rays remained and continued to concern the doctors as their cause remained unknown. This inflammation should have been resolved after being on steroids for over a month, so my pulmonologist suggested I get a lung biopsy. With a lung biopsy, a cardiothoracic surgeon takes a sample of lung tissue, which is analyzed by a lab to determine a diagnosis. The biopsy would require a three- or four-day stay in the Intensive Care Unit (ICU) with a chest tube. My pulmonologist and surgeon discussed whether I should have an open lung biopsy, which means a large incision, or a video assisted thoracoscopic surgery (VATS) procedure, which uses a small incision. Thankfully, they chose to go with VATS. The silver lining to having this procedure was that I had already met my insurance deductible for the year, so the biopsy would be like a medical vacation.

On December 9, 2011, I had the lung biopsy. There were no complications, and my recovery was normal. I was discharged home with oxygen, just as before. I remember being so excited to finally find out what was wrong with me. But alas, the results were inconclusive. For a time, I continued with the same treatment of steroids, antibiotics, and oxygen but was slowly weaned from all three. About three weeks after the biopsy, I found out I could return to work. I looked forward to returning to the predictable rhythm of regular life.

January 2nd was a Monday, and I knew only a few people would be at work because it was a recognized holiday. The quietness on the unit would allow me to sort through my email inbox and transition back into work in peace. I was excited about going back to work and couldn't believe that a supposedly simple procedure had evolved into a major health crisis that resulted in three months off work. I laid my clothes out the night before and had my lunch packed. I also made sure my car was full of gas. (Well, actually, Robert made sure my car was full of gas. He always knew how much I despised going to the gas station.) I woke up early and went to work that morning, happy to see the few faces that were there. That evening I came home and reported how well my first day back had gone.

The next morning, an intense pain in my lower left back awakened me. It hurt worse than labor. Every slight inhale felt like a knife stabbing into my back. The pain was so sharp I could barely talk, but I managed to wake up Robert and tell him I needed to go to the emergency room. He sprung out of bed, got dressed, and let our nephew and the big kids know we were headed to the hospital and that they needed to watch Rae Rae. When we got there, the staff immediately took me back to get a CT scan. I struggled to even get onto the gurney to go down to the imaging room. It was even more difficult to transfer from the gurney to the CT table and lay flat. Then, the techs wanted me to hold my breath off and on throughout the scan, which made the pain even worse. They finished the test and gave me some pain medication. The emergency room doctor came in and informed me that both my lungs were "whited out," which meant they were full of something. The CT image showed what looked like lots of fuzzy cotton flurries floating around my lungs. The emergency room staff notified my pulmonologist and admitted me to the hospital for ... you guessed it ... pneumonia.

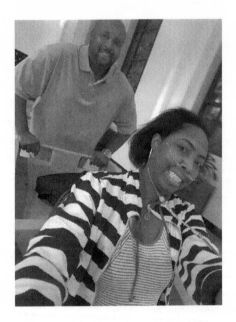

FOUR

We Is Pregnant Now!

I STAYED IN THE HOSPITAL about two weeks and was discharged home with antibiotics, steroids, and my newest companion, blood pressure medications. Apparently, prolonged steroid use was causing my blood pressure to rise. (I think the stress of being in the hospital several times for undetermined reasons was the real culprit for my increased blood pressure!) Eventually, I recovered from this case of "pneumonia" and went back to work in late February 2012. Everything was fine. No cough. No pain in my back.

Amid all this drama with my health, we had been set to close in November on the house we were building. Thanksgiving week, the bank told us they would not be able to carry out the loan because the losses we had sustained from our copier consulting business three years earlier were too much. This extended our time in the trailer. Looking back now, I'm convinced this apparent disappointment was divinely orchestrated. If I had been off work with a new mortgage in the books, it could have been catastrophic to our financial health.

Soon after I recovered and returned to work, we began working on house number two. We debated about whether we should build again or look for an existing home. We looked around and talked with our builder. Finally, we decided to build again, so we could customize a home to our specific needs and desires. However, before we signed the building contract, we looked at three homes on the market. We fell in love with one of them. It was in a great neighborhood and had all the bells and whistles we had selected for the home that had fallen through. Plus, it had some extras! Its list price was significantly higher than our budget, but the market was a little unpredictable, so we figured we'd give it a shot. Our Realtor cautioned us several times about how low our offer was and how much money the seller would have to bring to the table to make the deal happen. Still, we were confident in our offer and knew we could always find another house if this one didn't pan out. Before we put the offer in, I did a little research to discover the home owner's name. Immediately, I recognized the name as that of my pulmonologist. "There can't be too many people with that last name in Denton," I thought. At my next follow-up visit just a few days later, I asked him if his house was on the market. It was! His family had just built a house in nearby Frisco and needed to sell it. I told him Robert and I had looked at his house, loved it, and were probably going to put an offer in on it.

38

We put in our lowball offer, sat back, and waited. As expected, they refused our first offer and responded with a counteroffer, which was way out of our budget. We informed our Realtor that we were sticking with our lowball offer and proceeded to talk with our builder about building our home. While on vacation about three weeks later, I received a phone call from our Realtor. "If you're still interested in that house," he told me, "They're willing to sell it to you at your price!" Our answer was a no-brainer. Alas, we were moving!

I always wondered if my doctor sold it to us at our low offer price because he had almost killed me during a routine bronchoscopy (though it wasn't his fault). Maybe, though, it was simply a situation where he needed to get rid of the house. Either way, we came out on top.

Life settled into a pretty normal rhythm at this point. We moved into our new home on Mother's Day. With trailer life in the rears, we all appreciated our new space, especially the kids! Then in October of 2012, we found out we were pregnant. We had been trying to conceive but were surprised it happened so quickly, for it had taken us almost a year to get pregnant with Rae. We found out we were having another girl and decided to name her "Londyn." We were thrilled and grateful.

Raelyn's pregnancy had been relatively easy. I had worked up until my due date, hadn't gained an excessive amount of weight, and hadn't had any nausea or morning sickness until the doctors started my epidural in Labor and Delivery. For the most part, Londyn's pregnancy was following the same route. We assumed this would be a normal, easy pregnancy and delivery. It turned out our assumptions were wrong. Very wrong.

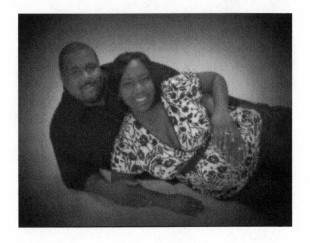

FIVE

"You Don't Look So Good"

EVERYTHING WITH LONDYN'S PREGNANCY went well until I reached about thirty weeks. It was National Nurses Week, and as a member of the leadership team at the hospital where I work, I helped deliver dinner and gifts to the night shift at 9:00 p.m. It was the first week of May. I was walking out to the parking lot at the end of the night and remember thinking there was no way I would make it to June 26th, Londyn's due date. I wobbled to the car and drove home. On the way I called Robert and told him the pregnancy was becoming too much. I didn't know if I was just tired because I was in my third trimester or if something else was going on.

The next week, I had an appointment with my obstetrician (OB). When I walked through the door, she told me I didn't look so good. "I don't feel so good," I replied. They did the test where they wrap the straps and monitor around my belly to check the baby. Londy was fine, but my own shortness of breath was concerning. My OB referred me to my pulmonologist, and after assessing me, he admitted me to the hospital and placed me on oxygen. Neither doctor wanted to do x-rays or anything invasive that could harm Londyn, but they were thinking that maybe pneumonia had reared its ugly head again.

I stayed in the hospital for about a week and celebrated Mother's Day 2013 there. They placed me on telemetry and monitored Londy and me frequently. Robert had gone to Colorado with his parents, so my mom came up to help with the kids and to be at my bedside. When I returned home, I was on oxygen again. My breathing did not improve, and I was fearful my breathing issues and the oxygen I was on could be harming Londyn. So, I made an appointment with my OB. It was the day before Robert and my eighth wedding anniversary. Like déjà vu, I walked through the door and my obstetrician told me I didn't look so good. Again, I replied, "I don't feel so good." Even wearing portable oxygen, I found it difficult to breathe. I couldn't even lean back in a chair, so they could monitor Londyn and check her status. My obstetrician sent me straight to the women's emergency room.

I sat in the lobby for a short time before they got me back to a room. When they moved me back, the first thing they did was check my oxygen saturation. It should be 95% or more, but mine was in the 70s. The nurses and respiratory therapist began frantically scurrying around the room. They told me to change into a gown and get into the bed. Simply trying to undress exhausted me, and I had to take breaks throughout the process. Remove one arm. Rest. Remove second arm. Rest. But, I did it. I put the gown on and crawled into the bed. They slapped a high-flow oxygen mask on my face and started making rapid-fire phone calls. I could hear the whistling from the oxygen blowing in my nose. It was coming out so fast and so loud. I overheard the nurses saying things like "ICU" and "emergency surgery." All I knew was I felt a whole lot better with that oxygen blowing in my face.

After about 30 to 45 minutes, my oxygen saturation was over 95%, and the staff informed me I was headed to the ICU. The only catch was they hadn't done this before with a pregnant woman. The women's department was on one side of the hospital and the ICU was on the other. They would need to send women's department nurses over to the ICU to check Londyn throughout the day. They transferred me to ICU and informed me of the plan of care. I was 33 weeks pregnant, and the goal was to get me to at least 35 weeks. They still didn't want to do x-rays but assumed I had pneumonia again. They treated me with antibiotics, low-dose steroids, and breathing treatments to get me through the day. Thankfully and remarkably, Londyn seemed to remain unaffected by all my drama. Her heart rate was good, and she was reactive.

The nurses were extra kind and attentive. I think they were scared to have a pregnant lady in the ICU. The dietary staff came through often and asked if I had any cravings or wanted anything special to eat, and they always kept my snack supply up to par. I was doing a little better but still got winded when I walked from the bed to the bathroom. After a little over a week in ICU, they decided to do an x-ray. I was requiring more and more oxygen to maintain a 95% saturation rate, and even though Londyn seemed unaffected, it still wasn't good to need so much oxygen.

The x-ray showed there was something inside my lungs. They weren't whited out as before, but there were definitely flurries in them, and the bases of both looked like honeycomb. It was coming up on Memorial Day weekend and my birthday. My OB was going to be out of town. However, the team decided they needed to take Londy, so they could treat my pneumonia aggressively. My OB met with her team and the on-call doctor, who was the most experienced in the bunch and the one who would do my planned emergency Caesarian section (C-section). The on-call doctor came in and explained everything that was going to happen and why it was necessary to do the C-section soon. They had other scheduled C-sections already planned but would get me on the schedule for the next morning.

Robert and I were confident in the doctor's skill set and explanation, and we agreed with his decision to deliver Londyn. We didn't recall the doctor informing us of any potential negative effects of the seemingly standard birthing procedure. He explained to us that the team would to do a C-section, so they could treat me aggressively. As far as the pneumonia went, in my head I thought they were going to take the baby and then do some type of lung cleaning while they were messing around down there. Mind you, I was low on oxygen and may not have been thinking clearly, but Robert heard the same information and had the same idea in his head.

The next morning was May 25th, my birthday. The doctor came in early and said they had to move a few other cases around, but I would be going back to the operating room around noon. I called Robert, my mom, and my best friend Tamara to alert them that baby girl was coming that day. Robert made it up to the room and the doctor made one final round before surgery. I remember the doctor standing in front of us in his surgery scrubs, hat, and boots, arms crossed in front of him. "We planned for this," he told us. "We coordinated with all the teams, and I've prayed about it. It's in the Lord's hands now." I agreed but didn't realize just how serious it was about to get.

The nurse and anesthesiologist came in to prep me for surgery and gave me a little happy juice. Robert and my mom walked behind my stretcher as the team rolled me down the hall. I remember the nurse telling Robert he couldn't come into the OR because it was an emergency situation. He would be able to see Londyn afterwards in the nursery. He gave me a kiss on the cheek, and the nurses pushed my bed through the large silver doors. I looked up and saw four different teams of people around the room. All gowned, gloved, and masked. There was a Neonatal Intensive Care Unit (NICU) team, what looked like an x-ray team, and others who were helping with the surgery scattered around the operating room. I still had my wedding ring on. The nurse saw it and asked me to remove it. I couldn't because my hand was so swollen. I honestly don't remember if she removed it or not. Soon after, I fell asleep.

Londyn was born at 12:22 p.m. on May 25, 2013. She went straight to the NICU. Apparently, when they started surgery, my respiratory status significantly dropped. They hurried to get Londyn out, so they could close me up and provide me with proper oxygenation. They came out and told Robert the baby was going to the NICU and I would be headed to the ICU. The doctor later told him I was in a grim state and had been placed in a coma. The prognosis was not good. The doctors and nurses were happy that Londy had survived but thought I would probably die as a result.

It was very stressful ... the plan was to save the baby 'cause they didn't figure Lia was going to make it. I was asked to go get the insurance policies, and they would help me get through this process of leading into death for Lia.

After walking out of the hospital to go get the insurance papers, it just hit me. I was trying to be happy that Londyn was born, but at the same time, I was grieving that my wife was dying. I went home like they asked me to, picked up the insurance papers, and was gonna head back to the hospital ... and it was at that moment that I was like, "I'm not taking these papers back. I don't want to force this action." I wanted to go back to the hospital and just continue praying and let my family know what was going on. So, I didn't take [the insurance papers] back.

I got back to the hospital, and they asked where the papers were. And I said, "I didn't bring them." And I didn't bring them because I felt that God was going to move in our direction. He was going to help Lia to live. He had brought us so far—everything we'd been through before to get to this point—to give birth, for my wife to die right after. So, I called Pastor, and we went to praying like crazy.

—Robert Young

SIX

I'm Alive, But What Happened?

I OPENED MY EYES AND SAW a white board with a baby's picture on it. A cute baby. I looked down at my legs and reached to feel them. "Great, I have legs." I felt for arms. "Check, arms are here." I turned my head slightly, but I couldn't move and there was a sound of metal when I tried to open my mouth. I didn't know what was happening. I knew I was in the hospital, but I didn't know why or what had happened. My mom was at my bedside, and I pressed the call light for the nurse. She came in and welcomed me back to the world. She explained to me that I had delivered a baby, been in a coma, and currently had a long, flexible plastic tube running from a ventilator through my mouth, down my throat, and into my lungs to help me breathe. I had been intubated. I made a motion to write. She handed me a pen and paper. All I could think of was that I had bought Beyoncé tickets as a push present for myself. The concert was supposed to be the Saturday after Londyn's

48

due date, about a week from delivery. In my head, if she told me I had delivered a baby, then I also had a concert to get to. I scribbled the letters "B E Y" on the paper several times in what looked like three-year-old handwriting. She finally figured out I was writing "B E Y" for "Beyoncé." When she said, "Beyoncé," I lifted my hands up in the air and mumbled, "Tonight, tonight." She thought I was crazy. She couldn't believe that a woman who had delivered a baby, almost died, and been in a coma for seven days didn't ask for her husband or baby first. No, I asked for Beyoncé. She giggled and informed me that I would not be going to any Beyoncé concert tonight. I may have seemed strangely preoccupied. The reality was I had great seats and didn't want them to go to waste. Someone needed to use those tickets!

AS I SAW IT

She survived that ... and the very first word out of her mouth when she survived the coma was, "Beyoncé."

—Robert Young

Robert was in the NICU with Londyn and came over quickly when he heard I was awake. I was so happy to see him. He slowly filled me in on everything that had happened. I spent most of the day trying not to be anxious and begging the respiratory therapist (RT) to extubate me (remove the long tube from my lungs). He checked on me every hour, and I hovered over my call light like a contestant on Family Feud when he wasn't in my room on the dot. My nurse kept asking me if I wanted morphine to ease my discomfort. She encouraged me to be patient and not anxious. Through writing, I told her I didn't want the morphine and that I would be less anxious if I had the tube out of my throat. After a full day of pleading and promising to do breathing treatments or anything else necessary, the RT finally called my pulmonologist. I heard him tell my doctor that my numbers were a lot better and I was getting pretty anxious and wanted it out. My doctor agreed to discontinue intubation, and the RT prepared me for extubation.

I didn't know what to expect. It was a quick "1, 2, 3," and he pulled this long tube with attached ruler-like metal pieces from my mouth. The tubes were full of mucus and saliva, and all I could think was, "Wow, all of that was in me?" He removed the sticky patches from my face and placed me on oxygen. I coughed and took several deep breaths. The amount of mucus the human body can produce is truly amazing!

I was on the road to recovery. Nurses, respiratory therapists, and x-ray techs stopped by my room to say hello and help me sort out what happened during Londyn's delivery. Many of them had tears in their eyes as they shook their heads in disbelief that I was alive. I had beaten the odds. I was not supposed to be here. I had some good ugly cries that day.

Throughout the afternoon, I slowly regained my voice, although crackly, raspy, and with a somewhat more country drawl. I had heard about people who had been in comas and had woken up with British or Spanish accents. That didn't happen to me. I got country instead.

Staff started coming in like clockwork as soon as they heard I was awake. The social worker asked if we needed any financial assistance. She left the room crying after hearing my story. I couldn't eat anything but ice chips, and I had a hankering for Popeyes, which was odd because during my entire pregnancy, I couldn't even smell fried chicken without feeling nauseous. The speech therapist and dietician came by to assess my swallow. They advanced me to a mechanical diet, which meant I could eat solid food if it was pureed or chopped into small morsels. I was so disappointed when I saw my bacon and eggs cubed and in little mounds on my plate. It was not what I had expected. I was soon advanced to a general diet, and my thoughtful nurse ordered me a summer fruit tray. The first thing I ate was sweet watermelon and plump, juicy strawberries.

I had to learn how to walk again. The physical therapist (PT) and occupational therapist (OT) came to help me get up for the first time. I started by sitting on the side of the bed and gently pressing my feet into the floor to wake them up. After a few minutes, we attempted to stand up. I couldn't. I had no strength in my legs and had lost so much weight. We waited longer and attempted again. I got up this time but felt very unsteady. My head seemed so heavy upon my neck, I rested it on my chest. I didn't have the strength to pull it up on my own, so I asked the PT to hold it up for me, so I could see. That one act of standing up had me winded. They helped me back into bed. The lactation nurse came in to help me pump breastmilk for Londy. I'm all about breastfeeding. I used to work in postpartum and helped many moms through this process. However, for seven days I had basically died, and my body had focused all its calorie usage on breathing and surviving. Producing breastmilk hadn't made the cut, and now there wasn't anything coming out of those dry hanging baskets. I was okay with that. As long as Londy got fed, we'd figure everything else out.

The world seemed brand new to me. I could taste every ingredient in ice cream, and fruit was juicier and sweeter than anything I could remember. The commercials advertising HD looked so vivid that the characters on the screen seemed to jump off the screen. A big track meet in Oregon was on TV, and I remember how amazed I was at the idea that these athletes were earning the title of best in the world. It blew my mind. What would it be like to be the best in the world? I looked around at my surroundings. Lying in a hospital bed with ice cream and fruit and breath in my lungs, I felt like I was the winner.

The next day Londyn was going to be discharged. She had progressed well in the neonatal ICU over the last eight days. Robert had gone shopping with his sister and found some preemie clothes. We were caught off guard by her early delivery, and the newborn clothes we already had swallowed her. She was only four pounds, five ounces. Robert got special permission to bring her into the ICU to visit me. She was about eight days old, and it was the first time I had seen her. She was so tiny and had a head full of hair. Even at her small size, she was too heavy for me to hold. Robert laid her beside me on a pillow. She was so tiny that it made me nervous. I played with her little hands and feet. Robert bundled her up and took her home where my mom and in-laws were waiting to help.

I continued to recover and became stronger every day. After about three additional days in the ICU, I moved to a regular room. My family and friends continued to visit. Robert brought me barbecue and helped me take my first real shower in weeks. I remember how he lifted me from the bed and carried me into the shower. I buried my face in his neck and breathed deeply. He smelled like barbecue smoke. That intimate moment is one I will always hold close.

It felt incredible to let the hot water beat over my back and shoulders, lather up with girly scented bath gel, and remove all the stickers and adhesive from my skin. Brushing my teeth with my electric toothbrush and gel toothpaste was the gravy on top. My nurse on my first night on the regular floor gave me a much-needed foot massage as she sang gospel hymns to me. This was definitely a new experience for me, and it felt so good! I had no pain from the Caesarean and was gaining the strength back in my legs.

Somehow Robert was balancing work, me in the hospital, and five kids at home. It was a crazy-busy time for him. My head was still a bit fuzzy about what had happened. It was almost two weeks after Londy's delivery when my coworker helped me realize I had been in a coma for seven days, not three days as I had thought. My doctors discharged me home a few days later. The last thing my pulmonologist said to me before I left was, "Don't get pregnant."

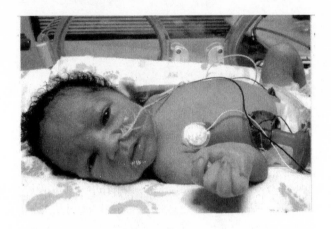

SEVEN

What You Talkin' 'Bout Doc?

IT WAS HARD FOR ME TO get into the routine with Londyn that was already somewhat established. We set up the Pack 'n Play in our room. Robert had bought a little white lace bassinet on wheels, which we used for Londyn throughout the day. I would get help lifting her because I was still quite weak. I would prop her up on a nursing pillow or set her beside me on top of a stack of pillows so that I could feed her. It took me a long time to shower, get dressed, and do morning activities. My mom stayed with us, which allowed Robert to work. Our church family, my work family, our soccer family, and our friends supported us through it all. They delivered food, came to visit, and prayed for us. The kids went often to their friends' houses or to my in-laws. School was out for the summer, and we were trying to save a little money by keeping Rae out of daycare. My sister-in-law would bring the kids back to the house during the day, and it would disrupt the routine I was trying to establish. I remember having a mini breakdown because there was just too much going on. I insisted that Rae return to daycare to promote some type of normalcy and to give us (aka me) a break during the day. On top of it all, the IRS had decided to audit us, and there was a gigantic pile of mail on our dining room table. But God's grace was sufficient, and somehow, we got through it all—audit, childcare, my health crisis—with strength I didn't always feel.

Londyn was healthy and was quickly making up for being born five weeks early. I was still on oxygen and had an occasional cough, which seemed to be allergy related. Raelyn was both excited and concerned the first time I was able to go upstairs to help her pick out her clothes and tuck her into bed. I hadn't gone upstairs in months, and this time it was only possible with my nasal cannula on.

I returned to work right before Labor Day. Life was back to normal. Raelyn was in kindergarten, and Londyn spent the daytime hours with a family friend while Robert and I were at work. She was still so young, and we didn't want to expose her to all the kid germs at daycare. My occasional cough became more frequent, but I chalked it up to allergies. Eventually it developed into something more intense, so I figured I should get it checked out. I went to my pulmonologist, who ordered me to get x-rays. The x-rays showed pneumonia ... again.

At this point, the pneumonia diagnosis was getting old. I'd had enough of it. This had to be something else. A healthy person should not have recurrent pneumonia like this. So, I went to the same pulmonologist in Dallas I had previously visited for a second opinion. He did several breathing tests and x-rays. Before I left that appointment, he told me my lungs had severe damage, and he was not going to experiment with my health. He projected that I might need a lung transplant. This was the first time anyone had uttered the word "transplant." He wanted to send me to the best respiratory hospital in the country for more testing and referred me to Denver, Colorado. He also gave me a signed and stamped application for a temporary handicap sticker, which, by the way, was the best thing ever!

I contacted the hospital in Denver to follow up with the referral, and after many calls between them and insurance, we were set to go to Colorado in late January 2014. We made travel arrangements, which included air, hotel, rental car, and oxygen. Robert and my in-laws would go with me initially while my mom stayed in Denton with the kids. Then for week two of my testing, my mom would come to Denver and Robert and my in-laws would go back to Denton with the kids. We flew to Denver. My breathing was significantly compromised even on the flight out. As the airplane began ascending, I felt tightness in my chest and was short of breath. I had to turn my oxygen converter up to its maximum output just to maintain some type of breathing function. We landed, and I was escorted via wheelchair to baggage claim. We got our bags and headed for the hotel suite, which would be home for the next two weeks. Because I wasn't a child, all my testing was considered outpatient, so we had to provide our own accommodations.

On Monday, I met with the team. They told me the plan of care and gave me a schedule of every test I would have to take. They conducted a thorough history and reviewed all the medical records I had sent from my many hospital visits as well as the lung biopsy results from 2011. I did every test known to man. CT scans. X-rays. PH probe. Six-minute walk test. Stress test. A bronchoscopy. You name it. I had it done.

The following Monday, Robert and I were scheduled to meet with one of the respiratory specialist doctors, who planned to tell us the results of all the testing and determine the plan of care. We walked into the small room. Robert and I sat on one side, and the physician sat on the other. He logged into the computer to pull up the images of my lungs. Rather nonchalantly, he informed me that I had scleroderma and non-specific interstitial pneumonia (NSIP). He said my illnesses had not been caused by aspirating water at a waterpark as I had originally suspected.

My first thought was, "What the hell is scleroderma?" He informed me that scleroderma was an autoimmune disease that had no cure and that can cause damage to internal organs and to the skin. It was unknown how you get scleroderma or NSIP, but they were related. There is usually not a family link, women get it more than men, and its onset usually occurs in people between 25 and 55 years old. It was very similar to lupus, sarcoidosis, and other autoimmune diseases. It was difficult to diagnose, but several factors combined to lead them to this diagnosis. My esophagus was slightly wider than normal, and I had some gastrointestinal reflux. I also had some symptoms of cold intolerance and Raynaud's (a condition marked by numbness of finger tips in response to cold temperatures), even if it was only in my right middle finger. My most significant symptom was pulmonary fibrosis, or scarring, in both lungs. Simply put, my body was attacking the healthy tissue in my lungs, which resulted in significant scarring. This scarring had reduced my lung volume from about 80% to about 34%. After rattling off all my symptoms and everything that was wrong, the doctor said I would most likely need a double lung transplant in my lifetime. He added that even when I get a transplant, they are only good for about five years.

My world began spinning, and I think I may have even blacked out for a few moments. I looked at Robert, my eyes wide open, and started to cry. My mind spiraled with questions: *What do you mean I need a double lung transplant? Do they even do that? I have a baby who's eight months old. Will I even be alive to see her fifth birthday? And what about Rae's 13th birthday, and Jasmine's graduation, and Telia signing her big scholarship for soccer? What about the other countless moments I haven't imagined yet? And what's the use of going through a transplant if I'm only going to live another five years?*

Then just like that, the doctor patted our shoulders and left the room. We sat there in silent shock, our minds racing with thoughts of what the future may or may not hold. One thing was certain: we had a lot of work to do.

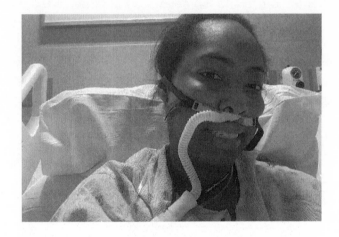

EIGHT

Going, Going. Back, Back.
To Texas, Texas.

THE PHYSICIAN'S FELLOW CAME IN and started talking to us more in depth about lung transplantation and scleroderma. There was a physician in Dallas who had trained in Denver. They were referring me to him to manage my care and transition onto the transplant list. The first things I would do upon my return home was to get steroid pulsing, an outpatient procedure in which high doses of steroids are administered via IV for two to four hours per day for a certain number of days, and begin taking immunosuppressive drugs in hopes we could get my body to stop attacking itself. I prayed the medication route would work and the transplant could be delayed or even avoided. Daily I praised God for His healing power and trusted Him to do His will, whatever that may be. I didn't want to have to go the transplant route, but if it meant improving the quality and length of my life, I had to consider it.

We left the doctor's office in Denver, picked up my in-laws, and told them the news. The car was quiet. I sat in the car while they walked into a store and called my mom and my best friend Tamara to tell them the news. The future was filled with so many unknowns, and this scared me. Robert and my in-laws left the next day and my Mom came out. I still had a few tests to do, and then we would go home.

I made it back to Dallas and did the three steroid pulsing treatments. The plan was to suppress my immune system so that my body would stop attacking itself and hopefully the damage to my lungs would stop progressing. In the meantime, I did a lot of research on scleroderma. I found a support group that met in Dallas and planned on attending. Scared to death, I went to the first meeting. For many people suffering with scleroderma, their skin is affected by the disease. Skin contractures are very common, and some patients with scleroderma have a certain look about them. Their mouths can be small, and their skin can appear tight. Sometimes the skin is so tight that it bends joints. After hearing the stories of these scleroderma survivors, I felt very fortunate that it had only attacked my lungs and not my skin, hands, or other internal organs. I hadn't heard from the doctor I was referred to in Dallas, so I followed up with him myself. Unfortunately, I had to call several times to get an appointment, but persistence paid off, and I finally saw him in March.

The pulmonology team did all the standard tests: six-minute walk test, Magnetic Resonance Imaging (MRI), CT scans, and breathing tests. I also met with the pulmonary hypertension clinic to determine if the arteries between my heart and lungs were affected by my condition. Thankfully, I did not show signs of pulmonary hypertension (narrowed arteries) or heart issues. The plan was to treat my symptoms to keep them at bay, which would hopefully prevent the scarring in my lungs from progressing. I remained on immuno-suppressants, steroids, and blood pressure medication and continued to meet with the medical team in Dallas every six to eight weeks. For the most part, I had hit a plateau. There was no change for several months, and I felt pretty good. Then when summer arrived, I started feeling a little worse. I experienced shortness of breath, and the Texas heat seemed to affect me. I also tired out very easily. The team instructed me to wear the oxygen at all times, not just with exertion as I had been doing. It was quite the sight when I returned to work after my appointment with my nasal cannula on and my oxygen tank on my shoulder.

Since my condition was starting to worsen some, the pulmonologist wanted me to begin infusions of an anti-cancer drug called Cytoxan to reduce the inflammation in my lungs. He referred me to a rheumatologist who assessed me and wrote orders for eight sessions of chemotherapy. It was a different type of chemotherapy than breast cancer patients receive and would not require hospitalization or cause my hair to fall out. For each session, I went to the infusion clinic, had an IV started, and sat there for four to six hours while the medication infused. It always gave me a bad headache and a little bit of nausea, but I was always able to drive myself to the appointment and back home afterwards. The chemotherapy had no effect on the scleroderma or my lungs. I didn't necessarily get worse, but I didn't get better either.

After completing the rounds of chemo, I revisited my pulmonologist. He was somewhat disappointed, as was I, that the treatments had no effect. The results from my breathing tests and six-minute walk were declining. He informed me he was referring me to the transplant team. He was going to continue to monitor me, but I needed to get on the transplant team's radar.

AS I SAW IT

Lia carried her oxygen tank with her everywhere. She would bring her tank to church ... but she kept coming. She kept praising God! She kept believing God, kept believing for a healing!

—Pastor Duane White

I met with the transplant team. We reviewed my history all the way back to 2011. They explained the qualifications for becoming a transplant candidate and what I would have to do to become active on the list. It was a little overwhelming and introduced Robert and me to a whole new world, one we would become very familiar with. There was a sweet spot in which a patient could receive a transplant. First, I couldn't be so sick that I wouldn't survive the surgery, and I couldn't be so well that I didn't need the transplant. No one could predict when I would need the transplant. It would not be a scheduled procedure.

Most importantly, someone would have to die so I could live.

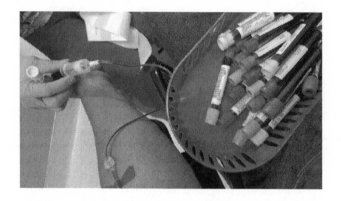

NINE

Can't Win for Losing

THE TRANSPLANT TEAM PROCEEDED with initial testing, which included determining my blood type, capturing detailed images of my lungs through multiple CT and lung scans, and testing for gastroesophageal reflux disease (GERD). These tests revealed that I had significantly high antibodies, some of which I had acquired from childbirth and from blood transfusions I received after Londyn's delivery. They explained to me that high antibodies make it harder—but not impossible—to find a match. I accepted the information but didn't think much about it.

Closer Look
Antibodies are the stars of the immune system, and their sole purpose is to attack foreign invaders in the body called antigens. Antigens include, but are not limited to, bacteria, viruses, and fungi. Antibodies are proteins that circulate in the bloodstream looking for an antigen to

attack. Everyone has and produces their own antibodies naturally. Women can get additional antibodies via pregnancy as the baby's blood mixes with theirs. People can also acquire additional antibodies via blood transfusions and organ transplantation.

This was my first introduction to Dr. Death. At first meeting, I immediately respected her intelligence and expertise. As a mother and hard-working professional, she was relatable to me. However, she never had anything good to say. Ever. She went over all my test results and informed me the team was concerned about the results of my swallow test. I had taken a test where I stood against an x-ray-type panel in the middle of the room. They provided me with a chalky drink and asked me to drink a little, hold it in my mouth, then swallow. As I swallowed, they moved the panel—and me—and took pictures of the substance going down my throat. The test's purpose was to see exactly what happens when I swallowed. According to this test, I had a mild case of reflux, which is common in scleroderma patients. Because of this, Dr. Death told me that before they would place me on the transplant list, I had to agree to not eat by mouth after the transplant. In my head, I assumed she meant for a certain time period and responded, "Okay. For how long?"

Dr. Death replied, "For the rest of your life."

Cue tears. Again, I looked at Robert sobbing, a million questions racing through my mind. He hugged me around my shoulders, and I buried my head into his chest. *What do you mean I won't be able to eat by mouth, ever? Do you know what a big part of my life food is? Every time we celebrate anything, food is involved. Every time we gather with friends or hang out with family, food is involved. Food is always involved!* Dr. Death obviously didn't understand my love affair with enchiladas, potatoes, and beef fajita nachos. She was out of her mind! Not eating was a key contingency. It may sound like a simple decision—life-saving organ transplant or eating—but, to me, it wasn't so clear cut.

I asked her a lot of questions about why I wouldn't be able to eat, how the feeding tube would work, and when it would be placed. Dr. Death explained that a PEG tube, which passes into the stomach through the abdominal wall, would be placed in me at some point after I was put on the transplant list but before I received the transplant. I would meet with a dietician who would order a certain "formula," which would be administered through the "button" via a tube and a bag. She explained that my reflux could cause me to aspirate food and liquids. If this happened and food or liquid got into my new lungs, it could cause infection, rejection, or pneumonia. Dr. Death offered several grim stories of patients who had broken the rules, eaten by mouth, aspirated, gotten infections, and died. I told her I would have to go home and consider this proposal. She sent in my nurse coordinator, who coordinated times for me to meet with patients who had required a PEG tube and/or no eating by mouth with their transplant. I met with them and learned that many of them were tube fed for only six to eight months. After praying about this decision, I finally decided I wanted to live by any means necessary. I informed my nurse coordinator that I understood and agreed to the requirements for not eating post-transplant.

The transplant team continued to follow me closely. My condition had plateaued ... again. It was getting harder to breathe, but I was maintaining. I was still commuting 45 minutes to an hour to work and working full time. I hauled my 12-inch oxygen tanks everywhere I went. I would load enough in the back of my Chevy Equinox to get me to work, through work, and back home. Robert or I would make the trip each week to my oxygen supplier in Irving, Texas to get 10-15 tanks at a time. It was not uncommon to hear the rattling of metal oxygen tanks in my car when we drove around town or hit a bump in the road. I had an oxygen converter at home that went up to six liters per minute.

As soon as I arrived home, I would put on my nasal cannula and go about my domestic duties. I coughed frequently, often to the point of losing my breath or vomiting. Water and peppermints or cough drops were my constant companions. Reaching my daily water-drinking goals was never a problem as the water seemed to keep the tickle out of my throat. Talking became difficult because I was constantly coughing or short of breath. I chose my words and conversations carefully and only spoke when necessary. It became extremely difficult to present information in front of my staff at work. I had to make sure I had water nearby and enough oxygen to last throughout the presentation. I couldn't whistle, yell, sing, or laugh heartily. All these things took my breath away.

Eventually I upgraded from the twelve-inch tanks to the big-mama thirty-six-inch tanks and had to use a continuous flow of oxygen versus receiving puffs of air. I also had a new oxygen converter at home that went up to 10 liters per minute. I quickly learned to choose my battles as far as what to expend energy on. There was no more going by the mall to shop after work and hiding my packages from Robert in the trunk of my car. Going out on date nights, with friends, or to events required detailed plans and calculations of how many tanks I would need and if I would have the energy to participate. Getting angry or upset resulted in shortness of breath and simply wasn't worth it. My personality became very laid back, especially with the kids. As long as no one was bleeding, it wasn't a big deal. Anything could be cleaned up or replaced. I didn't spend my energy on yelling or chasing after them, and I did my best to keep them organized and to teach them to do small things on their own.

I got so many looks whenever I went out and about. I could see on people's faces that they were trying to figure out why such a young person was wearing oxygen. I even had a woman lay hands on me in Macy's while Londyn and I were trying to shop. She acted strange and kept talking about "the manifestation." Honestly, she kinda freaked me out.

Throughout this time, Raelyn was very concerned and would often come to my side and just rub my back. She would tell me she was praying for me and wished I felt better. She wasn't the only one. This was about the time I really started to get concerned too. I began to ask

God, "Why me?" I mean, I had followed all the southern girl rules. I went to high school and graduated in the top of my class. I was even crowned prom queen! I went to college, graduated on time, and had a good-paying job lined up before graduation. I met a man, fell in love, didn't get pregnant before marriage, and married him. I attended church, prayed, fasted on occasion, and had a playlist of gospel music on my phone. I was a good girl, so it didn't make sense that this could be happening to me. At that time, I figured that's how things work with God—like a cosmic balance sheet.

For as long as I can remember, I had three fears. One was getting fat and not being able to lose the weight. Two was drowning. Three was getting a rare disease that had no cure. Thanks to steroids (which cause weight gain), the water park incident, and scleroderma, I had now encountered all my fears in one swoop. I would stand in front of the mirror with my oxygen on and just cry. But, I couldn't even do that right because if I cried too hard—good, ugly sobs—it messed up my breathing. I couldn't win for losing.

There were several times, maybe four max, when I thought about just ending it all. When I had to ask someone for help or had to mentally prepare my plan of attack before completing a simple task, or when I would hear Robert let out a silent sigh when I asked him to do just one more thing, I'd think about just getting out of everyone's way. When I had to turn down the kids' invitation to join them at the park, or when I had to sit in the car to watch Rae Rae's soccer practice because the air was too hot or too cold or too windy, I'd consider throwing up the deuce and finishing it all. I even thought about how I would do it. Option one would be jumping in a pool with an oxygen tank to weigh me down. But, I figured the tank would probably float, and I'd just be wet. Besides, we didn't have a pool, and jumping in my neighbor's pool to do the job would just be rude. Option two would be the carbon monoxide in the garage scenario. However, we had a lot of oxygen tanks and other chemicals stored in the garage. It would be just my luck that the carbon monoxide would activate some chemical reaction and blow the whole house up. Plus, we had everything but our cars stored in our garage. I couldn't fit a car in there if I tried. So, I guess I would suck it up, put on my big girl panties, and buckle in for the ride.

I thought about what the kids' lives would be like without me. I didn't want the girls to grow up without their mom. I didn't want Robert left alone to make all the decisions and to teach the girls girly things. Nope. Not today. I fought those feelings of despair by praying and by remembering what God had already brought me through. I also kept thinking God must have something incredible planned for my future. After all, why else would He have woken me up after Londyn's birth? I was still banking on my cosmic balance sheet, and I figured my payoff must be coming. Or so I thought.

TEN

Lookin' For Lungs

IT WAS THE HOLIDAY SEASON 2014, and at my quarterly visit with the transplant team, they explained that my condition merited going through the evaluation process and getting on the list. I was getting to the point to where I could get really sick really fast, and they didn't want me to be without options. Once I went through the evaluation process, (hopefully) got accepted by the team, and was placed on the list, I could ask to be made inactive if my condition improved or if I was going to be out of town for an extended time. Ideally, however, I would get on the list and remain on it until transplant. I began the evaluation process immediately after the new year.

The first part of the evaluation phase was a four-hour class, which covered everything transplant. In the class, we reviewed who was eligible to be a candidate for transplant, paying for the transplant, and private insurance versus Medicare and Medicaid. A double lung transplant was estimated to be a one-million-dollar surgery, at least. They told us the importance of family support and made us identify primary and secondary caretakers. We covered nutrition and diet while waiting for the transplant and after it was completed. The social worker talked to the class about the cost of medications, expenses which may arise that insurance would not cover, housing, transportation, and life after the transplant. She also emphasized the need to start fundraising immediately.

At the end of the class, my nurse coordinator handed me a packet with my appointments for the next two to three weeks. Most patients got their tests done quickly over a week's time, but because I was still working full time and conserving my paid time off, I elected to have my tests scattered over several weeks. The hospital was up the street from my job, so it was easy for me to get away at lunch or leave a little early to get a few tests completed. In total, I had twenty-one appointments, which included meeting with a cardiologist, pulmonologist, dermatologist, dentist, gynecologist, psychologist, and every other "-ist" known to man. I was scheduled to have scans I had never heard of in departments I never knew existed (and I'm a nurse!).

My mom came with me on one of the longest days ever. We had to shuffle from building to building, all day long. It was cold, and I was tired. Still, it was good to get this part out of the way, and I was glad my mom was there to hold my purse and my hand. I completed my tests and consults, and my transplant coordinator met with me to review the results. Thankfully, I was the perfect candidate with no other underlying medical issues. She planned on presenting my case to the board, who would then determine whether to accept me as a candidate.

The board met a little over a week later. Honestly, I felt I was a shoo-in because I wasn't sick (other than my jacked-up lungs and high antibodies), and I had everything they asked for: good insurance, family support, and a compliant attitude. During this process, numerous family members and friends supported and prayed for me. I regularly updated them on my status and where I was in the process toward transplant. Truthfully, I didn't think my current situation was that bad. I mean, I figured I could go through life carrying a small oxygen tank and making a few simple accommodations. I'd be fine. I even began to tell people that I really didn't want the transplant and asked them to pray for healing. I wanted to be one of those miracle stories where the person goes to the doctor and gets the worst diagnosis only to return weeks later and the illness had disappeared. I had played that scenario out in my head and believed God could do it. (I *still* believe He can heal people any way He chooses!) I imagined myself going to see the transplant team and Dr. Death coming in and saying, "Mrs. Young, we can't explain it, but we don't see any sign of pulmonary fibrosis. You're healed!"

But, that wouldn't be my story. I felt pretty sheepish post-transplant when I read about pre-transplant patients who had to overcome everything from weight loss or gain to extreme dental work or lack of family support to even be considered for the evaluation phase. There I was, with the opportunity basically given to me, failing to recognize it as the gift it was. Who was I to say to God, "Please heal me in *this* way. Thanks!"? Still, despite my presumptions and pride, God loved me, and He made a way.

My coordinator contacted me to say I was fully accepted as a candidate. They would put me on the list as inactive and let my condition determine when I would become active. She reviewed the United Network for Organ Sharing (UNOS) and the Lung Allocation Score (LAS). These two acronyms are very important in the transplant world as they determine where a patient falls on the list. The sicker you are, the higher your LAS. When an organ becomes available, the person with the highest LAS score gets the organ(s). Lungs are extremely difficult to acquire because they are often damaged in car wrecks or through the measures used to keep a person alive.

My high antibodies were another obstacle, a major one. There are several classes of antibodies. As it was explained to me, I had two classes that were super high. The range for these two classes were zero to one hundred; my scores were 96 and 78, so these specific classes were plentiful. Not only did my donor need to have my blood type, but he or she also needed to have these classes of antibodies present. Getting a transplant without matching antibodies could cause immediate or chronic rejection of the transplanted lungs. My body would see the new lungs as foreign and fight them off, which would cause rejection and result in the need for aggressive treatment or even death. Then, just to make things more interesting, the first year after the transplant is highly critical. Post-transplant patients are on a drug regimen, which includes immunosuppressive drugs that keep their immune systems from attacking everything in sight and a cocktail of antiviral, antifungal, antibacterial, and antirejection meds. This suppression of the immune system makes getting sick highly likely. In addition, patients take multivitamins and supplements to balance the chemistry in the body. Many patients experience rejection and/or some type of infection and do not make it past the first year.

I continued seeing the transplant team every three months. My breathing tests were stable at this point, surprisingly, but my six-minute walk test results had declined. The six-minute walk test is used to determine how far a person can walk and how much oxygen is required per minute to keep her oxygen saturation above 90%. I needed fifteen liters per minute and only walked 900 feet. Six months prior, I only needed four liters and walked close to 1500 feet.

It was fall, and I often had my mind set on doing things with the kids. Football games, soccer games, decorating, and going to the fair. However, the allergens in the air and my lack of energy kept me behind closed doors, drowsy on Benadryl with my oxygen cranked up. A simple walk from our bedroom to the kitchen often resulted in coughing fits and shortness of breath, and date night cancellations with the hubby were almost guaranteed. No sitting outside by the fire pit watching the girls play. No walking around the mall looking for a new comforter and a pair of cute joggers. I couldn't even move clothes from the washer to the dryer. Days like these made our decision easy. When my coordinator and transplant physicians suggested in October 2015 that I become active on the list, Robert and I agreed. We had prayed long and hard. We knew God was in control and would work everything for my good—whatever that looked like. I prayed for comfort and for peace and for God to restore all I'd lost while dealing with this illness over the past four years. I also began praying for the family of the donor who would give me the most precious gift—life.

It was official. I was waiting for a double lung transplant.

Robert and I informed our family, talked to the kids, and set up a GoFundMe account. I joined a Facebook lung transplant group and did a lot of research on current innovations in lung transplantation. I even researched what I should pack in my "go bag" for when I got the call. It felt like preparing for a baby. We made sure our phones were working and got a signal booster for the house. I informed the Unit Clerks at work that I was active on the list and asked them not to take any messages but to refer calls directly to me.

I prayed fervently and often, and I fasted from the trap music I enjoyed so much on my commute to work. Instead, I began playing gospel music the whole commute to and from work. It was my alone time with God and made a big difference in my attitude and feelings throughout the day. Being alone with God armed me for each day's challenges.

Robert and I stocked the pantry like it was Y2K and tried to keep up with laundry and toiletries. We informed Rae Rae and Londy's teachers and school administrators of our situation, so they would be ready if our parents began picking them up from school while I was receiving the ultimate gift. I bought 50-foot nasal cannula tubing, which allowed me to move about the house freely. Watching the kids play jump rope with it also made for good entertainment. I think they enjoyed hearing me yell, "Hey! Watch my cord! It's pulling my ears! Are you trying to kill me?" When they didn't know where I was in the house, they could always find me by following the tubing.

Robert and I both thought that this would be a good season to be active on the list. Let's be honest, people always die around the holidays. We selfishly hoped that some drunk college student attending the state fair, a holiday party goer, or a saxophone-playing non-smoker would have an unfortunate but timely death between October and January 1st. But ... it didn't happen.

I waited and waited for six months. Not one call. Not even a dry run. I began reading about being double (or dual) listed and researching other transplant centers around the country. There was Duke, Pittsburg, and even Houston. At my six-month checkup, I inquired about dual listing. I wanted to know my transplant team's opinions on the subject and if they thought it would be a good idea for me. The doctor, who had just transferred from a different center up north, and the nurse practitioner both cautioned me about the rarity of scleroderma patients even getting on many transplant lists to begin with. "Most transplant centers don't even place scleroderma patients on their list," they warned, "because of their specific symptoms and the disease process of scleroderma." I took their words as an admonition that I had better be happy and satisfied where I was.

So, I remained patient, but I continued to do my own research on dual listing, comparing the mortality rates of my current center with others in Texas and around the country. I was willing to go anywhere. At my nine-month checkup, I inquired about dual listing again. The nurse practitioner leaned in close to me as though he were giving me his social security number and said, "You need to get double listed ... like now. It's been nine months and you've had no calls. You need to broaden your pool of possible donors. Try Houston." When my coordinator came in a few minutes later, I told her I was interested in getting dual listed. I explained my reasons, and she agreed.

My center usually referred patients who wanted to be dual listed to a hospital in Houston that was a high-volume transplant center. My coordinator had a contact there and would file the necessary paperwork and be in touch when she was able to confirm an appointment.

After several emails and phone calls, I finally had an appointment in Houston. Robert and I would go in July to repeat the evaluation process for transplant at that facility. We would stay for a week. Again, we had to provide our own transportation, accommodations, and food. We found a facility that provided discounted housing accommodations for patients and families who needed long-term care or were receiving outpatient treatments. Insurance wouldn't cover oxygen in Houston, so we got as many tanks as we could from my local supplier and paid out of pocket for twenty tanks from a Houston supplier. We drove two cars on the five-hour trip to Houston. Robert and I were in one car and Jasmine, Robert's oldest daughter, and her friend rode in the other. Both trunks were full of oxygen tanks, and we were filled with hope that what hadn't happened in Dallas would happen in Houston. This was the first step in what we thought might be the break we needed.

ELEVEN

Houston ... I Have a Problem

THE EVALUATION PROCESS in Houston was almost identical to the one in Dallas. Thankfully, the Houston center was able to use the results from some of the tests I had done in Dallas. I met several other patients who had come from all over the country looking for lungs. Some were worse off than me, and some had diseases I had never heard of. Still, we were all united by one simple, profound thing—we all needed lungs. I completed my testing and met with the team prior to heading back home. They told me I was a great candidate but that my high antibodies were concerning. The team in Houston planned on presenting my case to the board and letting me know their decision. We returned to Denton and waited.

We thought about what being dual listed would look like practically. *Where would we live so that I could be within two hours of both centers? Would I just live by myself between Dallas and Houston or in Palestine,*

Texas with my Mom? Would I still work, or would I go ahead and take that disability my doctors in Dallas had been offering to write?

About a week later, I heard from Houston. They wanted to try plasmapheresis—a procedure in which blood plasma is removed, treated, and returned to the body—to reduce the number of antibodies and hopefully make me a better candidate. Pending the results of the plasmapheresis, they would put me on the list.

Y'all, I had to bug the scheduling coordinator like the chick on *Single White Female* just to get the plasmapheresis scheduled. She wouldn't call or email me back. I had questions about the process and wanted to know if I could get the procedure done in Dallas and just go to Houston for follow up. The coordinator finally called me back and informed me that the plasmapheresis had to be performed in Houston where they had a special lab and tests specific to patients with my condition. It had now been eleven months since going active on the transplant list, and we hadn't thought we would still be waiting for lungs, much less traveling outside of Dallas. We scheduled the procedure for the Tuesday after Labor Day. I would be there for two weeks. We rented a hotel suite close to the hospital this time, and it would just be Robert and me. Before leaving, we prepped meals for the kids and had special talks with Rae and Londy. I told them I loved them so very much and was doing all of this so that one day I could live, participate, and support them fully. During this time, Robert and I also had many heart-to-heart

83

"when you get your lungs" talks. I whispered countless prayers and shouted out more than a few too. I also cried plenty of big, ugly cries.

We made plans for our friends and family in Houston to visit and relieve Robert over the weekend. My best friend, Tamara, planned to come down to check on me as well. It was evaluation time at my job, and Robert was busy too, so we packed our laptops and planned to work in the afternoons and while I was receiving treatments. The treatments would be every other day and last for about four hours at a time. On Tuesday, the team in Houston would place a tunneled catheter (a tube about the girth of an ink pen) in my jugular vein with IV access ports coming out of my right chest wall, and I would start treatments on Thursday.

For the treatments, they would access my catheter, pull my blood out, spin out the plasma, and toss it. Then they would replace my high-antibody plasma with an artificial plasma and return the blood to me. I had read that the treatment made people feel cold and drained, almost like having the flu. I had prepared for this with an electric blanket and gloves, though I wasn't allowed to use the blanket as it was considered unsafe. They gave me warm blankets instead. As planned, they placed the port in me on Tuesday.

That night, my dear sweet husband wanted to be intimate. That experience somehow dislodged my catheter, and it began to leak. I woke up the next morning with blood from my chest on my gown, pillows, and sheets. I sprung out of bed, found some towels, and started applying pressure. It wasn't working. I called the number on my discharge paperwork, and they told me to come in immediately. Robert drove me back to the hospital feeling guilty about his lead role in the previous night's extracurricular activities. The doctors and nurses placed me in a room in the day surgery area and attempted to stop the bleeding. Of course, I didn't tell them the real reason why it started leaking. In all my tests and appointments and procedures, this was the only time I was vague about anything. "I don't know what happened," I said innocently. "I just woke up, and it was leaking."

The hospital ended up admitting me to a semi-private room. Tamara was coming to relieve Robert, so he could go back to Denton and be with the kids. My roommate in the hospital was an elderly lady, and as I was wheeled into the room, her family was discussing how she hadn't slept in three days. The room was huge. My bed was by the window, and the bathroom was near the entrance door—past my roommate. The nurse had to put several extensions on the oxygen tubing, so I could reach the bathroom. It was horrible.

They moved my roommate out, and I asked them to move me to the bed closer to the door and bathroom. They moved me, and I had the room to myself until about midnight, which is when they rolled in a new roommate. Everyone was talking loudly and carrying on as though it were twelve noon! I was in my own personal hell and all over a few moments of intimacy with my husband.

The oozing stopped, and an x-ray verified that the catheter was still in place and patent. They transferred me to the apheresis center for my first treatment. All the blogs and articles I had read were true. Once they started removing my blood, I got extremely cold. My fingers turned blue, and not just the middle finger on my right hand this time. After the treatment, I felt drained. All I wanted to do was sleep. They discharged me from the hospital, and I rested the remainder of the weekend. I completed the treatments over the next week, and we returned to Denton. Prior to leaving, I had my blood drawn, and Houston planned to call to let me know if the plasmapheresis had effectively eliminated the high antibodies and if, subsequently, I could now be placed on their transplant list.

I was exhausted … but hopeful.

TWELVE

Hitting the Wall Face First

I FELT HORRIBLE WHEN I GOT home from Houston that Friday. I was so tired and felt nothing like my typical 90% self. I went to work on Monday and did the bare minimum. When I left work, I called my Dallas coordinator from the car and told her I felt bad and needed to come in. She told me I needed to get my monthly labs drawn anyway, so I could just get them done and drop by the office. That night, I tossed and turned. I couldn't get comfortable. I got up to go to work Tuesday, but I kept coughing and had to take breaks to catch my breath while getting dressed. I had no energy and called in sick to work. I couldn't hold my arms up long enough to comb the girls' hair. I couldn't walk the ten feet to the bathroom. And I couldn't talk because it would make me winded and exhausted. I called my coordinator and confirmed that I would be in her office by noon on Wednesday. That night, I started mentally preparing to go to the doctor the next morning. It was going to take a mountain of effort just to get out of the house, but I had to do it.

Robert and I woke up, and I attempted to get the girls ready for school. I got so out of breath doing the girls' hair that I asked Robert to crank my converter up to 10 liters per minute and bring me a fresh portable tank. I turned the portable tank up to 15 liters per minute and crowded both nasal cannulas into my nose. Sitting on the edge of the bed, I closed my eyes and took several deep breaths. I could feel my heart pounding. Seven-year-old Rae held my hand and said, "I'm so sorry you're having a bad morning. It's probably good that you took off work. I love you and can't wait for your lungs to come." Londy, three years old at the time, threw her head into my lap and just hugged me.

"Damn!" I thought. I hated that their childhoods were littered with these images. I kissed each girl, and Robert took them to school. Slowly I inched my way to the garage and waited for him to come back and pick me up. He helped me load up, and we headed to Dallas.

The valet at the hospital met me at the car with a wheelchair. I was panting and couldn't get enough air in. He whisked us up to the transplant office and back to a room. My coordinator was there, and the look on her face confirmed what I already knew—I didn't look good. She called in another nurse, and they set me up to attempt the six-minute walk test and a test called spirometry to assess my current lung function. I kinda rolled my eyes and thought, "I really can't breathe right now. How am I supposed to do this test?" She placed a pulse oximeter on my finger to get my oxygen saturation, and it indicated I was in the low 80s. The nurse cranked up the oxygen and gave me a full facemask. My saturation slowly crept up. She kept turning it up … 12 liters, 15 liters, 18 liters, 20 liters, 25 liters. Finally, I reached 95% saturation. She walked out of the room and grabbed my coordinator. My coordinator walked in and told me I had just bought a ticket to the emergency room.

The emergency medical technicians (EMTs) came to the office with their stretcher and equipment. I had returned to the room with Robert and was sitting on the exam table breathing in the oxygen on high flow. My coordinator gave the EMTs the scoop on my condition. They started hooking me up to the heart monitors and switching me over to their portable oxygen. One EMT asked me what organ I was on the transplant list for, and I replied, "Toes." I mean, really? I'm sucking on all this oxygen and you ask me what organ I'm needing replaced?

The paramedics took me to the ambulance, and we travelled about 0.2 miles to the main hospital across the street. Robert met me there, waited until I got settled, and rushed to Denton to pick the kids up from school. I called my mom and Tamara to let them know what was going on. Robert called my job to tell them I had been admitted.

I started thinking that I was in that window the doctors had told me about years ago—that time in the disease process where my lungs were like, "Mic drop. I'm done. Can't expand anymore." I couldn't fake it until I made it. I had arrived. I was sick. This could be my calhl.

AS I SAW IT

I'm still amazed by Lia's ability to see good and humor in everything that would make most cry. Today as the paramedics were preparing her for transportation on the stretcher, they went over her vitals and a few other questions. One of the questions was, "What are you having transplanted?" Note that Lia is on a crazy amount of O2 since they are trying to keep her oxygen saturation up. Lia tells the paramedics her toes are being transplanted and had the biggest smile on her face. Then she turned to comfort me ... my perception? I married a beautiful, awesome, strong but crazy woman ... but damn, I love her!

—Robert Young

The emergency room doctors, respiratory therapists, and nurses rounded on me. They assessed me, drew blood for lab tests, and performed breathing treatments. They ruled out pulmonary embolism and all viral and bacterial infections. They saw a little fluid around my heart and attributed that to the slight increase in pulmonary hypertension. They thought that

I was having a "flare" as a result of having all the fighters in my blood wiped out with the plasmapheresis.

I was enjoying the oxygen. My mom showed up in what seemed like an hour from when I called, even though she lived about two-and-a-half hours away. After waiting in the emergency room bed for seven hours, my penthouse suite was ready, and the staff transferred me to it around 8:00 p.m. The room was huge. It was on the twelfth floor, had a 70-inch flat screen television, a pull-out bed, and a beautiful view of the Dallas skyline. Robert returned to the hospital, and my mom spent the night.

The next day, I met Doogie Howser from the internal medicine team. The team rounded on me twice a day and managed my overall case, which included an assessment, a review of my history, and communication of their plan of care. Then the advanced lung disease team came and did the same thing; their reports then provided guidance for the respiratory therapist. The transplant team also did regular rounds to inform me of my status on the list and my new LAS score. My latest shenanigans had moved me up to number one on the transplant list for my blood type. My patient care techs and nurses were amazing.

When I was first admitted, I was still able to walk to the bathroom with my oxygen tubing extended. However, just a few days later, I was no longer able to get out of bed without assistance. I used a chariot-like contraption to stand and roll into the bathroom to use the toilet and shower. It was crazy how quickly my condition worsened. In one week, I went from fully ambulatory (able to get up and move on my own) to limited mobility to a bedside commode and bed bath. The slightest move or smallest amount of talking induced coughing, shortness of breath, a racing heart rate, and a significant decrease in my oxygen saturation.

Robert and the kids visited often until flu season began and children 12 and under were no longer allowed to visit. Londy seemed scared of all the tubes that were hooked up to me. Raelyn was worried. She asked a lot of questions, and I had to try to remain positive and answer them on a kid level. My mom stayed with me 24/7, and my in-laws moved into our home in Denton. This allowed Robert to have help with the kids and attempt to work. My friends and co-workers came to visit as well. Many of them didn't realize just how sick I was. They brought food, flowers, and gift cards. Tamara and my friend Jessica decorated my room. I could tell I was declining, and as October approached, I was seriously banking on getting my blessing soon.

I likened this journey to a pregnancy, and I was a first-time mom in her thirty-ninth week and sixth day of pregnancy. I had gone through all the stages of wondering if I should get pregnant, hoping to get pregnant, getting pregnant, and preparing for the baby. Even still, no new mom is ever fully prepared! That was me, ready for labor and delivery … ready for this journey to reach its destination. It was "go" time! I had my trap music blaring and my "Phelps" face on. I wanted to see my baby and get back to those pencil skirts and high heels.

I was ready to get the call that my new lungs had arrived.

Day and night, Bible verses and gospel songs set up camp in my head. "Do not be anxious about anything, but in every situation, by prayer and petition, with thanksgiving, present your requests to God. And the peace of God, which transcends all understanding, will guard your hearts and your minds in Christ Jesus ... And my God will meet all your needs according to the riches of his glory in Christ Jesus" (Philippians 4:6-7,19).

Every verse I had ever learned as a child or read as an adult came flooding back as I tried to hold God's truth higher than my current reality. "Now to him who is able to do immeasurably more than all we ask or imagine, according to his power that is at work within us" (Ephesians 3:20).

At night, I put in my earbuds and listened on repeat to the gospel playlist on my phone. I listened to the lyrics and prayed silently for healing. Each time Travis Greene's "You Made A Way" came on, tears streamed down my face, and I wondered if I really was going to come out on the other side of this mountain alive.

I had faith and felt God was going to push me through the finish line. I had accepted that I might just die from this but believed deep down that no matter what, I would *still* win. Whether I died that day and met my Savior Jesus face to face or received a transplant and lived another twenty years, I would *still* win. This was a turning point for me. I had thrown out the cosmic balance sheet that had once driven my decisions and my perception of God, and I started speaking life into the situation.

One of my pastors, Kris White, had just preached about the importance of having a positive mindset. I started visualizing my girls and me on the beach, Rae's sweet-sixteen party, and Londyn's fifth birthday. I began making plans for when I had pushed through this, for when life returned to its beautiful, ordinary normal. I praised God for the victory He had already won even when all I could see with my physical eyes was the battle in front of me. Then, in the wee hours of the morning, I heard a preacher on television speak about asking God for something *BIG*. No more sick, wimpy requests. Instead of saying, "Lord, send me lungs so that I shall at least live to see Londy graduate from high school," I started praying *BIG*. "Lord, heal me and bless my life. Redeem the time our family has lost while dealing with this sickness. Restore every detail of our lives to a level of health and abundance we've never known before! Allow my journey to be a testament of faith to the masses. Let those lungs be perfect and last longer than these doctors could ever have estimated. Let me tell this story to my children's children's children."

I talked to Robert and told him that I planned on making it, but if I didn't, he was going to be a rich man in every way—spiritually, emotionally, financially. I told him to tell the girls I tried my absolute best, and I did all of this for them. I told him to get his Corvette, and I forbade him to play "Going Up Yonder" at my funeral. I gave him strict instructions about how I wanted to be cremated and my ashes stored in a blinged-out vase. I wanted a party or reception, not a sad funeral with people hovering over me saying, "She sure looks like herself."

While sitting in that hospital room, I asked Tamara to get me lined paper, so I could write letters to my girls. I wanted to tell them everything they needed to know just in case I didn't make it—everything from how to shave their legs to what to look for in a husband. But, Tamara couldn't find paper. In hindsight, I think that was God showing me the letters were not going to be necessary.

THIRTEEN

Shouting at My Mountain

THE PHYSICIANS CONTINUED to manipulate my oxygen equipment and plan of care. They tried different masks, CPAP machines, and BiPAP machines. Heck, they even tried Viagra. They threw in everything and the kitchen sink. The transplant team in Dallas contacted Houston because we hadn't heard from them since the plasmapheresis. As I monitored and participated in conversations and emails between the two centers, it became apparent to me that each center believed that how it practiced was right and best. In my opinion, this mindset prevents centers from sharing research and best practices. Patients get lost in the web while they try to make sense of it all. I'm convinced I went to Houston for plasmapheresis treatments that could have been performed in the very building where I sat in Dallas. The procedure did eliminate the antibodies, which was good, but the entire process was more frustrating and costly than necessary. The transplant team in Houston was taking my case back to their board for approval. If approved, I would be placed on their list, and if lungs became available, the Dallas team would transport me to Houston for the transplant.

Never the bearer of good news, Dr. Death informed me that the board in Houston had denied me. Yes, I was on my deathbed, and still, they denied me. Apparently, more recent labs drawn in Dallas showed that the antibodies had reappeared. Houston didn't want to risk transplanting me only to have my body reject the organs. I couldn't deny it—I was disappointed.

When Dr. Death first delivered this news, I thought, "Well, damn! All this time, money and stress for nothing! I really am gonna die waiting on these lungs." Then the usual vision of my demise went through my head, my commitment to having a positive mindset momentarily forgotten. The vision always involved the floor. In it, I was either eating a grilled cheese sandwich in the kitchen and passed out on the floor dead with said sandwich in grasp, or I was using the bathroom and fell off the toilet, bumping my head and dying instantly with matching panties and skinny jeans around my ankles. (The bathroom option was becoming a real possibility!) In this depressing daydream, my body headed straight to the funeral where somebody was playing "Going Up Yonder," even though I had clearly asked Robert not to let that happen. I had to snap out of it. Yes, the facts surrounding me were dismal, but deep down I believed the truth that God had not brought me this far to turn back now. I believed this truth was greater than the facts I could see.

AS I SAW IT

We went and spent a lot of time and a lot of money in Houston. To me, that was Lia's life line. We knew that in Dallas she only had less than a 1% chance of a transplant but in Houston it was 25%. So, for me, I hung my everything on Houston ... The day they were supposed to list her, they called and told us they were denying her. They wouldn't list her. It devastated me. I knew at that point things were already getting bad. I was dying inside when we first heard the news, but she looked at me and smiled and said, "Well, Dallas it is. We'll make it happen in Dallas." I'm looking at her thinking, "What is wrong with this lady? Either she crazy, or she's got tremendous faith."

—Robert Young

I remember my pastor, Duane White, posting a live video during this time in which he talked about shouting "Grace!" to the mountains and obstacles in life. He referenced these words from Zechariah 4:7: "Who are you, O great mountain? Before Zerubbabel you shall become a plain. And he shall bring forward the top stone amid shouts of 'Grace, grace to it!'" (ESV).

He asked his viewers to pray for me—to shout "Grace" to my mountain. So that's what we did. We shouted "Grace!" to the mountain and praised God for a victory we couldn't see yet.

Dr. Death made rounds on me often and always had this certain look on her face. It's difficult to describe. It was a look of attempted compassion but without any real faith that this situation was going to end positively. She always said, "You're so positive. That's good," in a tone that bordered on patronizing. I was placed on a machine that controlled the amount of oxygen I received and the force at which it was delivered. I was on 30 liters and not feeling well at all. Throughout the day, the time it took me to recover after any movement or coughing spell became longer and longer. My heart rate would rise to the 130s and my saturations would drop to the 70s, and it took me thirty to forty minutes to calm down and return to normal. These were true episodes. I would start coughing, become flush with heat all over my body, and signal my mom to turn on the fan and hand me my water. I would increase my oxygen, close my eyes, and take deep breaths. Next, I would get cold and signal for my mom to turn off the fan and pile blankets on me. Twice, the rapid response team—a team of nurses, respiratory therapists, and critical care doctors—busted into my room during an episode. I was on their high alert list.

Dr. Death mentioned I was progressing towards the maximum amount of oxygen and pressure that the current machine was able to deliver. The next step would be life support via intubation. To do this, they would insert a long tube down my throat and into my trachea then hook the tube up to a ventilator, which would breathe for me. The doctors made it clear they wanted Robert and me to go ahead and intubate right away. Doing so would allow my body to rest. However, it would also be risky because once I had been intubated, I might not be able to be extubated—or breathe again on my own without the ventilator. I called my coordinator to get her opinion. She said that being intubated would raise my LAS score but not drastically. In addition, whether or not I could be extubated was a huge gamble. We declined. The potential down side of intubation seemed to outweigh its benefits. After all, I had been active on the list a whole year with no lung offers. We didn't think a slight increase in my LAS score could make a big difference.

Dougie Howser popped in to see me one evening and told me there would be a new group of internists starting that night. "Don't scare them," he said. I was not compliant.

Around 8:00 that night, I became extremely short of breath and had another episode. I asked my mom to call for the respiratory therapist; he came in and adjusted the oxygen machine. My nurse came in as well. However, I was very agitated and could not catch my breath. I felt like I wasn't getting enough air in fast enough. They called a rapid response—everybody and his mama came to my room. They drew labs, assessed me, adjusted my oxygen, and decided I needed to be transferred to the ICU. They explained to me that my nurse had three to four other patients, and my condition required one-on-one care. I didn't want to transfer to ICU because it confirmed what I already knew—I was getting worse. I called Robert, who had just pulled into our driveway in Denton. "Robert, I'm scared," I told him. He came in what seemed like fifteen minutes. I looked at him and began to cry. I didn't know what was going on or why my breathing had become so sensitive. My nurse in the ICU held my hand and prayed for me. She told me I was a child of God, and He had plans for me. She said I had babies who needed me and stated that I would overcome. I needed to hear that.

On October 2, 2016, Robert teamed up with my nurse, my incredible co-workers, and our older kids to arrange a date night right there in the ICU where we renewed our vows. They covered my bedside tables with white sheets and laid out real plates, silverware, and wine glasses. They opened boxes of food from Bob's Steak & Chop House. There were steaks with all the trimmings, dessert, and wine. Robert and I had always wanted to go there but had never made it. Pastor Duane led the ceremony. Robert got down on one knee and gave me a new beautiful, big ring. And then, right there in the ICU, a saxophone player emerged from the hall playing some Luther Vandross. It was crazy! Robert never did anything halfway, and that night was no different. He wanted me to know that whatever happened, he would be right there beside me. He got his message across as only he could do.

The renewal was something I wanted to do for Lia. Behind the scenes, the doctors were telling me that she probably wasn't going to make it. If something did happen, I wanted to let her know that I'd be there for her, and I'd be there for the kids. That was a major thing to her—to know the kids are alright. I wanted her to know that I loved her no matter what's going on, and I was going to be there until the end.

—Robert Young

We had a lot of support. My staff from work sent someone to give me a manicure/pedicure and someone to the house to detail Robert's truck. People dropped food off at the house and sent toys for the littles. Most of Robert's clients for our copier consulting business were churches of various sizes all over the Dallas-Fort Worth Metroplex. They were all praying for us. I tried to update my GoFundMe page daily to keep everyone informed. People I didn't even know contributed to our campaign and were praying for us. I could feel the love and wanted to keep fighting and remain positive not just for my sake but for all those who were cheering me on. This victory would not be mine alone.

My situation was getting worse. I was becoming anxious. I could see my vital signs on the monitor and knew it was getting bad. I had never dealt with anxiety, and, honestly, I'd probably thought, "They crazy," when people told me they took "head meds" for anxiety. But, laying in that hospital bed, I came to realize that anxiety was real. God was forging me into a woman of tremendous faith, and I knew with unwavering certainty that God was going to work everything out for my good, for my family's good. In my mind and heart, I knew I didn't need to be anxious about anything. I believed God's promise that His peace would transcend everything I understood and stand guard around my heart. I had lifted my hands off the steering wheel long before. Still, when I was in the middle of a coughing spell and couldn't breathe ... when I felt my heart pounding and knew I needed to slow my breathing but couldn't ... when I had learned too much about my body and knew exactly what was wrong but could do nothing to fix it ... I started to get a little anxious.

Dr. Death and the respiratory doctors had several heart-to-heart conversations with Robert and me. They had explained three options, none of them great. The first involved the words "comfort care," which I knew was code for "hospice." However, the machine I was on couldn't be used at home, so I probably wouldn't make it home alive ... or out of the hospital parking lot. Comfort care would also take me off the transplant list. The second option was to intubate. The catch was that they would keep me on the life-supporting ventilator for up to fourteen days or until transplant, whichever came first. Option three was to just ride it out in my current state, which would likely conclude with a code blue situation and the end of my life. We chose to save my life by any means necessary and put off intubation for as long as possible.

I told Dr. Death that I understood intubation to be the start of a clock to the end of my life. I only wanted intubation as a last resort to extend my life. She placed her thin hand on my shoulder in an almost robot-like attempt to show she cared and said, "I know you're religious, but it's time to start dealing with reality." If I had had the breath and energy to gasp and cuss, I would have. I didn't, so I just smiled and thought really mean things about her. How dare she! Religious!?

This is the part in the story where it gets a little fuzzy for me. I remember that my mother and the respiratory therapist were in my room. We were talking about my O2 saturation level, heart rate, and blood pressure. I knew it was getting bad and asked my nurse to turn the monitor away from me so that I couldn't see it. Constantly watching it was making me anxious, and I was requesting anxiety meds around the clock. I remember posting on Robert's Facebook page, "Get here now!" because intubation was a real possibility, and I wanted to see him one last time, just in case.

We had a meetin' on a Sunday ... We knew that if she got intubated, she wouldn't be able to get extubated out of the coma. Once her lungs started getting assistance, they would give out completely. Dr. Death gave us 30 minutes to make a decision. We prayed, cried, and cried. At that moment, we made a decision that if she had to be intubated to save her life, it's what we had to do ... But if she ended up being intubated, we wanted to be together beforehand to share some words, vision for the kids without her.

—Robert Young

The next thing I remember is flashes of interactions with nurses, Robert, my work staff, and friends. My memories of this time are like slides in an old-school View-Master toy. I'd open my eyes and see something, then nod off. The next time I opened them, the scene would be totally different. I remember my stylist doing my hair with the help of my dearest friends Tamara and Jessica. I remember doing sign language and writing on a whiteboard to communicate.

The doctor came out and said Lia was awake and talking. I said "really?" I didn't believe her. I came into the room. They were asking Lia questions, and she was trying to answer. The doctor even pulled up sign language on her phone to try to communicate with her! So, since we both learned the sign-language alphabet in our fifth-grade class, I was able to communicate with her!

—Tamara Russell, Lia's best friend

I remember my staff from work and my pastors surrounding my bed and praying for me. I remember Jessica, wearing a beautiful yellow shirt, talking to me, and I remember my high-school classmate crying while she held my hand. I held her hand and told her to stop crying because it was all going to work out. I guess I looked pretty awful.

Later on that [Sunday], I was just devastated. I got home, laid in the bed, and was trying to put together the words to tell the kids Mommy's not going to make it. After about an hour of just lying in the bed trying to think of the right words to say to the kids, God hit me with a word—to find an alternative to what was happening in Dallas. I wish God spoke to me like in the story of Moses. That's not how God talks to me. It's normally through a dream or an idea ... when I act on it, something happens great. And when I don't act on it, something negative happens to me. So, when He told me to find an alternative, I got up that second, grabbed my laptop, and went into the kitchen.

My mom was in the kitchen washing dishes at 11:00 p.m. I set my laptop up, and the second I turned my laptop on, the other word from God was, "I've been waiting for you to take control of the situation." That's one thing I'd never done as a husband; I'd never taken control of this situation. With Lia being a nurse and being so active in research, I'd just stood behind the scenes and supported her. But the second God said He'd been waiting for me to take control of the situation, I turned my laptop on. To this day, I don't know what the email said, but I wrote out an email and sent it to 30 or 40 hospitals around the country and one in Canada.

The words, I still don't know what they said, but they were pretty powerful. Those words were definitely from God. So, I sent the email out, waited about 20 minutes and started to follow up with the hospitals I'd emailed. I spoke to a doctor in Canada who told me three hospitals I should follow up with. One was Duke. One was Loyola Marymount, and the other was Johns Hopkins. Even though she told me to do that, God sent me a different direction. For some reason, He told me to look up the University of Maryland, which I had never heard of and never been to. I looked this hospital up, and low and behold, they had a transplant doctor who used the same process as the group in Canada to save a lot of people who were going through the same thing that Lia dealt with. So, I sent the email to them, called them, asked to speak to Dr. Iacono, the world-renowned doctor who works with scleroderma and lung transplants. The lady answered the phone, and I said, "I need to talk to Dr. Iacono."

She paused like, "Who in the world is calling to speak with Dr. Iacono ... at 11:30 at night?"

So, I said, "Tell him Robert Young is on the phone." I know I'm just a nobody to him, but I felt something in my spirit when I asked to speak to him and said Robert Young was calling.

She paused, I asked her for her email 'cause she didn't say she'd connect me. I told her I'd like to send her the email I had just sent him. She gave me her email. She read it and told me to wait about 10-15 minutes and not to hang up. During those minutes, I'm copying and pasting and sending the email to about 20 more hospitals, just trying to see if anyone would hear my cries. She got back on about 15 minutes later and said, "Mr. Young, I want to pray for you right now." She prayed that one of the doctors would help us. She said, "I printed off your email and delivered it to the transplant doctors who are here tonight."

I said, "Thank you. I'm moving on to the next 20 hospitals." About 20 minutes later, I get an alert on my computer that I got an email. I was seriously thinking it was one of those junk emails saying I had won a flight to Tahiti or Hawaii. I wasn't gonna look at it, and something told me to. I looked at it, and it was one of the transplant doctors at the University of Maryland. He had reached out to me and said he wanted to see if he could even possibly help save Lia's life.

He promised me he'd call me the very next morning, bright and early. The very next morning is when Lia had really gotten sick and had to be intubated. And so I get the call to go back to the hospital. I go back, and she had already been intubated ... I already knew that if she got intubated, nine times out of ten she wouldn't be able to be extubated. So, I didn't get a chance to talk to her before intubation. To me, that was just devastating. Dr. Death walks into the room the second I get there, pats me on my shoulder, and is telling me, "We had to move forward. We agreed yesterday the process was to intubate her and a few days later take her off and let her expire ..." When they took her off, it would be about 20 minutes before she passed.

Another doctor (the "good" doctor) comes in and says to me, "Your wife is 38. She's too young to die. If there's anything we can do to try and prolong her life, I'll do it." She goes, "I'll be back." Meanwhile, I waited all day for the doctor in Maryland to call me back. He never did. About eight hours later, the "good" doctor came in with a stack of papers and folders and everything. When she turned the corner and came into the room, I already knew she was probably coming to say we needed to move forward.

"Mr. Young, I need to talk to you," she said. My face went from bad to worse when she said that. She goes, "I've been on the phone for the past eight hours with Dr. Iacono from the University of Maryland."

—Robert Young

The next thing I remember is Robert telling me I was going to Maryland. I was so confused. I'm all about travel, and Robert and I had a list of places we wanted to go. But I was a little preoccupied and couldn't figure out why in the hell I was going to Maryland. Were the crab cakes *that* good?

AS I SAW IT

I was the only one in the office, doing overtime …. While sitting there, the phone rang, and when I answered, Robert introduced himself and said with a shaky voice, "Please help me save my wife." He confessed his love for Lia and started explaining her condition. He said this [transplant at the University of Maryland] is the last resort. Chills went all over my body … and tears came to my eyes …. I had never heard love expressed the way Robert did for Lia, and I wanted Lia to live.

I said, "Mr. Young, how fast can you have all her records sent to me?" Then I printed out the records ... and delivered them to the doctors who were there. I said to them, "You all must help her."

—Talibah Anderson, former
 Transplant Administrative Assistant
 at the University of Maryland
 Medical Center

Closer Look
(Robert's Email from October 17, 2016)

My name is Robert Young. I'm calling around trying any and everything that I can do as a husband and dad to help save my wife's life. We live in the U.S. in Dallas, Texas where my wife has been listed for double lung transplant for close to a year and a half. The underlying issue for the need for transplant is scleroderma that attacked her lungs. She is an RN and the Assistant Director of Nursing for a large pediatrics hospital in Dallas. My wife Lia Young has been in ICU here for a month now. She is in need of a transplant quick but has high antibodies, so she has not been considered for a donor match since being listed. She's 38 and the mother of 5 with 2 (a 3 and 7 year old) from her womb. I've read your bio and saw that you and your research team have done some "high risk" transplants and have been successful. Please share any info that may help us extend her life. Anything that may help. Is there any way we can double list her in Maryland or any other hospital that utilizes the transplant program that you and your team have brought to light in recent years? Any help is greatly appreciated. She is in desperate need of lungs. We are willing to relocate immediately if there is any hope. We need her, so if there is any way to help, please hear our cries.

—Robert Young

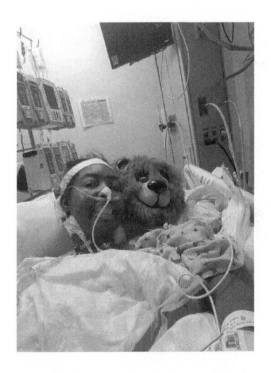

FOURTEEN

I'm Leaving on a Jet Plane

MY FRIEND AND FORMER CO-WORKER, Elilta, was at the foot of my bed. It was still dark outside. My nurses gave report to these other nurses who were suited up like a flight crew. I just smiled and nodded back off to sleep. My bed was moving and there was a line of nurses and doctors standing along the wall in the hallway outside my room. Was I dead and this was my *Soul Train* line to heaven? I nodded back off.

I woke up. I saw the ceiling of the room. One of those flight-crew-looking nurses touched my hand and said, "Lia, you are in a plane on your way to Maryland to get a transplant. We gave you some medicine to help you sleep and not move. We're almost there. Go back to sleep." I dozed off again. Then, I felt my bed move again. I heard an ambulance in the distance and was told I was about to be transported to the University of Maryland. The air was cold, and the roll from the plane to the ambulance was a little bumpy. They put me in the ambulance, and we sped off. I listened to the crew talk about a wedding and the apple beer that was on tap. I dozed off again.

AS I SAW IT

[The doctors in Dallas and Baltimore] had worked out all the insurance details. That was definitely a miracle. The medical flight was going to be $228,000. They wouldn't take a check. It had to be $228,000 verified funds.

Lia flew on a medical flight, and there were so many doctors on the flight me and my daughter couldn't fly with her, so we had to take a commercial flight.

—Robert Young

When I opened my eyes, I was surrounded by people in pink scrubs and hats. I felt the urge to cough and did. When I coughed, blood spewed from my mouth all over my chest. I couldn't move my arms, but I started motioning with my eyes to my chest. I tried to use sign language, but it clicked that I was no longer in Texas and Tamara wasn't here. I wanted to make sure someone besides me noticed what just happened. *Did anybody else see this?* They put towels on my chest and under my chin. One of the nurses got my attention and said, "Lia, you have a tube down your throat. It is very important. Do you know how important it is?" I nodded yes. "You're not going to pull that tube out, right?" I shook my head no. "Okay. Then I won't restrain you." I gave a thumbs up and nodded back off.

AS I SAW IT

[My daughter and I] got to the hospital about an hour after Lia arrived, and they told me she's in shock trauma ... This is something I'd never seen before and never want to see again. They told me she was in room 7, so me and my daughter run into room 7, busting through the doors. She was covered head to toe in blood. I thought we were going in for a lung transplant. It looked like she'd been shot. I thought they'd passed Lia through the ER and someone had shot her! "No, no, no," they said. "That's her lungs."

—Robert Young

The next time I woke up, I was clean and neat in a room. There were tubes everywhere, and I couldn't talk. I pushed the call light, and my respiratory therapist and nurse came in. They filled me in on where I was and what was going on. I was in the Lung Rescue Unit at the University of Maryland Medical Center in Baltimore. I needed pain medicine and my nurse offered some. I wrote on the whiteboard, "NO MJ." He looked at me funny then giggled. He got what I was trying to say: "No ... Michael Jackson ... don't kill me."

A nurse practitioner came in and explained that now that I was stable, the goal was to get me on the transplant list in Maryland. I was on ECMO (a form of respiratory life support), which would hopefully buy me some time until I could be transplanted. That day and night I went in and out of consciousness.

AS I SAW IT

After Lia arrived, we reviewed all the tests she had had in Dallas, assessed her physical condition, and formally presented her to the lung transplant selection committee to place her on the lung transplant waitlist.

She was a high-risk candidate (being on ECMO, having scleroderma, and especially having high pre-formed antibodies). However, with Dr. Iacono and me as strong advocates, the committee agreed to formally accept Lia as a lung transplant candidate.

—Si Pham, MD, former Surgical Director of the Lung Transplant Program at the University of Maryland Medical Center

Robert and Telia visited, and I used my phone to keep up with the outside world and paper and pen to communicate. The next morning, the nurse practitioner entered my room along with a social worker. They had folders in their arms. The nurse practitioner told me they thought they had a potential donor and needed me to sign the papers to get on the list and accept the donation. I almost fell out. I was so excited. I had received some pain medication and was afraid I might be delirious, so I asked her to call Robert and explain it to him. I texted him, "Possible donor ... Get here now."

AS I SAW IT

As soon as they had stabilized her, they put her on the list, and within four hours, they had a donor.

—Robert Young

They contacted Robert and began preparing me for surgery later that day. I was so happy and filled with anticipation. Later, the medical staff informed us that the heart patient had to have surgery first, so my transplant surgery would be the next morning.

AS I SAW IT

Curtis would be mad as all get out at the driver [who hit him] but thrilled to be a real life "angel hero" to all the organ recipients. He was a blessing in my life, and even on our worst days, I thanked God for the opportunity of being his mother and providing him opportunities to see the world in a more positive way ....

The tears still come pretty easily sometimes, but I know that is good for me as I grow and go through this grieving process. I am just so incredibly blessed by the knowledge that despite Curtis' earthly struggles he has been

118

such a huge blessing to so many because of his death. I continue to believe this was all part of God's plan for him (and me), and I cannot find fault with, nor do I plan to argue with God! And I know without a doubt Curtis would be thrilled by our decision to donate his organs. He would probably say something to the effect of, "No brainer mom. I won't have much use for them where I am going."

—Lois Yerrick, mother of Lia's organ
donor

The doctors had to fly somewhere to evaluate the lungs, harvest them, and bring them to Maryland. I remember hearing the helicopter when they arrived and Robert and Telia saying, "Your lungs are here." The anesthesiologist gave me some happy juice, and I went to sleep.

AS I SAW IT

Lia's double lung transplant was not a typical double lung transplant. Because she was on ECMO and had pre-formed antibodies, it required a lot of coordination. A donor team flew out to get her lungs and had to time it so the lungs would not be removed from the donor before we were ready at our home hospital. Another team performed the plasmapheresis in the OR while I was operating on her. The plasmapheresis (which took about 1.5 hours) had to be finished before we could implant the donor lungs, and we did not want the donor lungs to sit outside the body too long. The operating room was full of people, and there was a lot of pressure to get things done in a coordinated and timely fashion.

—Si Pham, MD

I woke up. Robert and one of the doctors were there. My stomach and chest hurt so bad, and I couldn't stop rubbing them. I looked up and mouthed to Robert that my stomach hurt. He smiled and said, "You got lungs." I looked at him like, what you talkin' 'bout Willis? He said it again, "You got lungs!"

AS I SAW IT

In the 11th hour, over and over and over and over and over, God kept doing it! He kept working behind the scenes.

—Pastor Duane White

I motioned, "When?"

He replied, "Yesterday." I burst into tears. I couldn't believe it. It had really happened. This wasn't a dream.

After the surgery, Lia looked at me and she goes, "Seriously, why is my stomach so sore?"

And I was like, "You have lungs."

She goes, "When? How?"

"Right now," I said. That's when the ball-fest started. We both just started balling.

She was the worst case they [University of Maryland Medical Center] had ever seen. They said if they had seen her before she got there, they wouldn't have believed they could do it.

—Robert Young

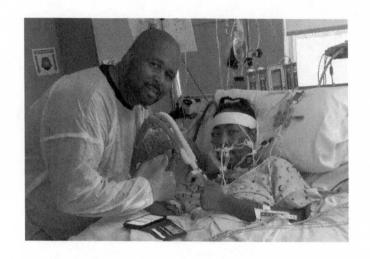

FIFTEEN

Blessed and Highly Favored

RECOVERING FROM A DOUBLE LUNG transplant is not easy, nor fun. I had five chest tubes, IVs in both arms, a nasogastric tube in my nose for feeds, a urinary catheter, a nasal cannula for oxygen, and ECMO tubes running from my right jugular to the top of my head to beyond my feet.

AS I SAW IT

Lia remained on ECMO after the transplant and continued with plasmapheresis for another five days. Many things could have gone wrong, especially bleeding, the transplanted lungs not working, or infection due to the prolonged ECMO and plasmapheresis. But it all worked out well. It was truly a miracle.

> I have been doing lung transplants for more than 26 years and have never seen one that worked out as well as Lia's. Much credit goes to the infrastructure and dedicated personnel at the University of Maryland Medical Center. It is one of the few places in the world that can provide such complicated coordinated care.
>
> —Si Pham, MD

Every morning started the same. Between 3:00 and 4:00 a.m., the x-ray tech brought the portable x-ray machine into my room and took x-rays of my chest. It was quite the task to maneuver the large, cold, metal board past all my tubes to my back. I laid on the board and held my breath as the tech took the picture.

Around 7:00 a.m., my nurses would give report to each other. They would come in and ask me how my night went, and we'd set goals for the day. Around 8:00 a.m., various members of the transplant team would come through—a Fellow or Resident, the nurse practitioner, the charge nurse. Then my physician and all the people I had seen earlier would stand outside my room and discuss my case. I always tried to turn my television down and listen in. There were issues with my left lung not expanding. We did several bronchoscopies at the bedside, and I was given frequent breathing treatments around the clock. We also tried a BiPap ventilator, but eventually I had to return to the operating room. I had a blood clot, about one liter in volume, lodged between my lung and rib cage. They removed the clot, placed an IVC filter in my groin, and gave me an additional chest tube. For the first few days, I received additional plasmapheresis treatments to suppress my immune system. It made me very cold, and I wore gloves and warm blankets during the process. They used a lift to hoist me out of bed and into the chair for treatments. It was a little scary—imagine your entire body being scooped up and lifted about four feet off the bed and swung over to a chair!

I spent the rest of each day working on breathing, surfing Facebook, and visiting with my nurses and techs. Around 8:00 or 9:00 p.m., I would get a bed bath, which was the worst. I'd get so cold as I log rolled from one side to the other. After the bath, they would lotion me up and apply lidocaine patches to my back and under my breasts to dull the pain. I had a clamshell incision— a perfect line under my breasts—and it was the main source of my discomfort. My other source of pain was my right shoulder. I don't know if it was gas or something else, but it hurt. Fortunately, warm packs, lidocaine patches, and hydrocodone 10mg made everything better. It was difficult for me to sleep. I don't know if it was the pain or medications keeping me awake, but I was often wide awake when my nurses and techs came in to perform routine vitals or breathing treatments throughout the night. Robert and Telia visited during the day and went home after Halloween. My friend and co-worker, Sherry, relieved them.

After about two days in the ICU, the physical therapy department informed me I was going to walk. Mind you, I hadn't walked since Dallas, almost a month before, and I was not excited about this goal set before me. But, I knew I had to do it and was told the physical therapist assigned to me was exceptional. So, surrounded by an incredible team, I attempted to get up and move. They placed the mother of all walkers at my bedside and raised the head of my bed up. I inched my feet off the side of the bed, and they maneuvered my chest tubes, IVs, oxygen, feeding tube, and ECMO. Anytime I moved, one or two ECMO technicians had to be present to manage the tubes. They affixed a gait belt to my waist, and I took some slow, deep breaths. I had lost a ton of weight and muscle tone and was very anxious about standing up. I assumed my legs would be like jelly. I grabbed the walker and stood up with a "1, 2, 3." I looked around but couldn't will my legs to take a step. I asked to sit back down and determined to try later. A few hours later, I stood up and took a few steps. Even though it was only a few steps, I felt a great sense of accomplishment. The next time I stood up was easier. With my gloves on and Beyoncé blaring through my phone, I walked to the entrance of the ICU and back to my room. It was the first time I had been outside of a hospital room in over a month.

Robert returned and began to work on securing housing for himself while I was in the hospital and for both of us once I was discharged. He couldn't spend the night with me in the ICU. My room was the best on the block. Displayed on the wall were an 8x10-inch framed family photo and a beautiful picture Telia had drawn. A Glade Plug-in kept my room smelling fresh and non-medical. I still wasn't eating, desperately needed sweet tea, and wanted to try the crab cakes Maryland was so famous for. They allowed me to have four ice chips—yes, only four—every hour. I asked if they could freeze some sweet tea and let me eat those. The answer was "no."

Finally, I had the opportunity to do a swallow test. This would determine whether I would be able to eat or would be on the PEG tube plan as mentioned months earlier by Dr. Death in Dallas. They took me to take the test, and thankfully, I passed. Immediately, I asked Robert to bring me some good sweet tea. One of Robert's high school classmates had a sister, Amber, who lived in Baltimore. We made contact, and she and her husband brought me cans of mandarin oranges. I was so thrilled to feel that sweet juice burst in my mouth!

I spent about two or three weeks in the ICU. Several of my chest tubes, one of the IVs, the feeding tube, and the urinary catheter were removed, and I transitioned to a stepdown unit, which was designed to prepare me for discharge to the home-tel. Robert had secured housing for us at a Microtel Inn & Suites about seven minutes from the hospital. The gift of gab and all those business classes he had taken had paid off as Robert made fast friends with the manager of the hotel and got the room for just $35 a night. Robert had set up the kitchen and adjusted to the extended-stay life while I was recovering. The social worker and coordinators had told us we would probably have to stay in Baltimore for at least six months and possibly up to a year. In the back of both of our heads were questions about how we would manage our family during this extended time in

Maryland. *Do we move the kids? Do we commute back and forth? Do we rent an apartment in Baltimore? Where do I work? Will my nursing license work in Maryland, or will I even be able to go back to work?* We had a lot of decisions to make.

Most of the teaching I received happened in the step-down unit. My physical therapists and occupational therapists visited me twice a day. They helped me sit, stand, walk, and climb stairs. It blew my mind how hard it was just to use the bathroom. Standing up from the throne felt like a controlled fall. They slowly and sneakily removed the bedside commode. Then, the walker inched farther away. Slowly, I became more and more independent. The dietician came through and discussed my diet after the transplant, and Robert and I had a full two-hour class on my medication regimen. The nurse entered my room with a University of Maryland duffle bag full of medicine, a blood-sugar monitor, and a blood-pressure cuff. She went through all the medicines, explaining what each was and why I needed to take it. She had me walk through each medication and place it in my mammoth-sized pill box. I also had to write my meds out on a medication record. I had to update this record as my medications changed and bring it to all clinic appointments.

It was mid-November, and Thanksgiving was right around the corner. I hadn't seen my kids since October, and I missed them. Video calls were just not enough. I wanted to hug and kiss them. The team prepared me for discharge. I was doing so well with PT that I wouldn't need to do outpatient rehab. I would have a home-health nurse come to the home-tel, assess my PICC line (an IV inserted into my upper arm that ends in a large vein near my heart), and teach me how to administer my antibiotics through it. I would need to have weekly blood draws and clinic visits. They warned me to use hand gel and extreme handwashing, stay away from crowds and sick people, take my meds, and keep my wounds clean. I was discharged the Tuesday before Thanksgiving, November 22, 2016.

We met the home-health nurse at our home-tel the night of discharge. She changed the dressing on my PICC line and taught me how to administer the antibiotics, which were in little tennis-ball shaped devices. I ate a piece of homemade cake that one of my prayer warriors had sent overnight, drank a cup of milk, and nodded off. Later, I woke up, my head nestled on Robert's chest. We hadn't held each other in months, and it felt so good to be in his arms. This had been a crazy ride, and he stayed by my side through it all. Wow, he really loved me.

I remember Robert telling me how surprised he was every time other men came up to him and said how amazing they thought it was that he had stayed with Lia through everything she went through. Robert said he didn't even know how to respond in these conversations. To him, that's simply what husbands do—they stick by their wives and their children. That's what real men do, and that's what Robert did.

—James Jackson, Robert and Lia's friend

The next morning, I had to do my meds all by myself. It took me over an hour to get it all right. I slept a lot that day and was still having some cold intolerance. Poor Robert was burning up because I had set the thermostat so high. My legs and feet were more swollen than ever before. I couldn't even wear shoes, and my feet hurt when I walked. Robert went out and purchased me shoes a size bigger than my normal size, and they still wouldn't fit. I resolved to wear fluffy house shoes.

My family was coming on Thanksgiving Day, and I couldn't wait. We woke up Thanksgiving morning and had a delicious lunch with Amber and her family, who unofficially adopted Robert and me during our time in Baltimore. Amber's brother, Jeff, was a classmate and close friend of Robert's. They lived in Glen Burnie, which is about 15 minutes from Baltimore. They visited me in the hospital and supported us like family in a place where we didn't know anyone. We left their house and headed an hour-and-a-half away to Philadelphia to pick up the family. The kids ran to my arms when they saw me. They looked so different, and I'm sure I looked different to them too. This was the first time in her life Londy had seen me without oxygen. We played all weekend. I told them how I was feeling and the plan for the rest of my stay. I explained that I was going to try to be home for Christmas, but it was highly unlikely. We drove up to Washington D.C. and visited the Martin Luther King, Jr. monument, and they returned home that Sunday.

I continued to manage my care from the home-tel. My walking got better, and I could take showers, do my hair, and even cook a little without getting tired. My legs and feet were still swollen. My doctor put me on Lasix to reduce the swelling and told me to wrap my legs in ace bandages and elevate them. I did as was told and freaked out when I woke up one morning to see that the swelling had traveled from the bottom of my feet to my waist. Everything was swollen. Thankfully, a boost of Lasix resolved everything.

Christmas and the new year were approaching, and Robert and I knew I would not be home for the holidays. We arranged for him to go home and be with the kids. Tamara, my mom, and my brother would fly out to be with me. Amber and her son, Ian, brought a Christmas tree and ornaments to the suite. We decorated it and hung all the Christmas cards we received around the room. It truly felt like Christmas.

The University of Maryland sent the media team to our suite to film my story and followed me with their cameras through a clinic visit. They use my story on their website, and because of that video, I've had many pre-transplant patients contact me to inquire about my experience.

Robert, the kids, and my in-laws came back to Baltimore after the new year. We went back to D.C., toured the Smithsonian, and ate some soul food. I was so happy to be alive and with my family and was getting the itch to go home. I was thankful my physician in Baltimore and his team agreed to accept me and saved my life, but there was no way I could move my family to Baltimore. There had to be a way to manage my care from afar. I started pleading my case to go home. I had a follow-up appointment with the cardiothoracic surgeon, who assessed my incisions and told me I was doing great. He also gave me way too many details about how the surgery was performed and how adamant he was about making sure my nipples were aligned correctly when he sewed me up. I asked him about going home and told him I had to be home by March 4th, Rae Rae's birthday. He thought about it and said I would probably be able to go home in February, but I would have to drive … no flying. With it being flu season, flying with potentially sick people would put me at risk. We decided to have our car shipped to Baltimore, so we could drive back.

The next week we moved out of our home-tel suite into the basement of another adoptive family we had met through networking and social media, Emmett and

Marilyn. We were so thankful for them! Texas doesn't really have basements. Storm shelters, yes. Basements, no. So, when our friends offered their basement and Robert replied, "yes," my mind went immediately to scenes from the movie *Kiss the Girls* with Morgan Freeman. You know, one light in the center of a room with concrete walls. Cold. Large rats. A trickle of water creeping down the wall. A dirty mattress on the floor and instruments of torture strewn about. Thankfully, it was nothing like my vivid imagination. The basement was like our own apartment, and the family was so welcoming. We were able to attend church with them and eat at all the places the locals go. We stayed there during our last month in Baltimore.

During that last month, Robert and I spent our days planning our next move, arguing with one of our insurance companies (they still haven't paid up!), and catching up on Netflix. We signed up for real estate classes, I gave grad school serious consideration, and I decided to write a book. I also wanted to be an advocate and inspiration for other patients who were going through the transplant process.

It was getting difficult to manage our family from afar, and I was antsy to get home. My final bronchoscopy was scheduled for February 6, 2017. Immediately after, we planned on hitting the road for Texas.

Our car was already packed and ready to go as we headed to the hospital that morning for my bronchoscopy. After the procedure, I took a little nap. Later that evening, after hugging and thanking our adoptive family, we hit the road. We knew it was going to take two days to get back to Texas, approximately 1,400 miles. We stopped in every major city along the way—Nashville, Memphis, Little Rock. We spent one night in Bristol, Virginia and one in Bryant, Arkansas. I've never been so happy to see the Texas flag at the state line in Texarkana. I almost cried. I loved seeing the cows, horses, open fields, and even I-35. So many construction projects had been completed and new ones started. Everything looked brand new. I had been away from my home for six months.

When we made it to Denton, our first stop was Kroger. We got a few items for home and a jug of sweet tea for me. Our pastors lived in our neighborhood, so we swung by their house next. I hadn't seen Pastor Kris in over six months. We hugged and cried and hugged some more right there in her driveway. Then we drove around the corner to our house, which was decorated with a "welcome home" sign and balloons. Our pastors and church interns had decorated the house and left goodies for Robert and me. The kids had made signs and posted them in the bedroom and all over my bathroom mirror. It was almost time for Rae Rae to get out of school, so we jumped in the car and went to pick her up. Robert was never one to sit in the pickup line. Instead, he always walked in to check Rae out, and she always waited for him in the office or lobby. That day I walked into her school, and she lit up with surprise. She grabbed me and hugged me, and the office staff started crying. Rae had taken on a lot while I was sick—burdens and responsibilities few children know—and I was so thankful to be home, so thankful I would get to see her grow up. We picked up Londy from preschool. Her response to seeing me was the same as Rae's. Mommy was home!

During all those months in hospital rooms, I listened countless times to a playlist of gospel songs on my phone. The first song on the list was "Blessed and Highly Favored" by the Clark Sisters. In it, they sing these powerful words: "He brought me through hard trials. He brought me through tribulations … Back was against the wall … He heard my cry and rescued me … Don't take for granted that we are here today. Just know that we're blessed and highly favored."

Deep down, I always believed these lyrics described me, that no matter the outcome of this trial, God was looking out for me. But now, back home with my girls, my mountain flattened and a future possible, I knew more than ever that I was blessed and highly favored!

SIXTEEN

Living Our Best Life

TRANSITIONING BACK INTO the many roles I play was challenging. Getting a lung transplant is lifesaving, and I wouldn't trade it for anything. However, in reality, a person trades one set of problems for other challenges. I can breathe and am able to do all the things I couldn't do before the transplant, but it comes at a cost. I take approximately twenty pills a day (and will for the rest of my life). For the first six months post-transplant, I had to give myself LOVENOX shots in my abdomen daily to prevent blood clots.

I was also a little anxious and hypervigilant about not getting sick. We had hand gel and wet wipes in all locations where I would be: my purses, cars, kitchen, bedroom. You name it; there was gel there. To this day, I wear a mask when I fly, and, for the first year, I wore one in all public places. The kids couldn't have live virus vaccines during the first year post-transplant because it was a threat to me. The kids gave me the evil eye at their pediatrician's office when I said they couldn't get the nasal spray flu shot. I continue to get my blood drawn every two weeks and do breathing tests regularly (and will do so for the rest of my life). I've read blogs about incidents where the post-transplant medications were thought to cause mood swings and personality changes. Fortunately, I haven't experienced that, as far as I know.

The medications I take are for a lifetime and all have side effects. Tacrolimus, an anti-rejection medication, causes my hair to thin and fall out. This was an important piece of information I didn't know beforehand. It was alarming to watch my hairline recede and my hair go from shoulder length to about one inch all over. It's coming back now, but the texture is completely different. Prednisone is a necessary evil that causes weight gain, high blood pressure, and hyperglycemia (aka diabetes). I was a slender 150 pounds when I returned from Baltimore but gained fifty pounds within eighteen months of the transplant. My breasts went from a manageable size D to an overwhelming and cumbersome F. I had tremors in my hands in the early months post-transplant, which made it difficult to pick up meds, do my hair, or write. And all the meds I take can potentially cause cancer, damage kidneys, and make me subject to sunburn.

But hey, I'm breathing!

My first year post-transplant was stellar. I showed no signs of rejection or infection. Robert and I traveled and did all the things I couldn't do pre-transplant. We relished every moment. Gladly, we returned all the oxygen tanks and equipment to our oxygen supplier. Robert and I got our real estate licenses, and I started working on my Master of Business Administration degree. I traveled back to Baltimore and had a perfect check-up. The first time I walked up the stairs in the house, I celebrated, and I took a selfie the first time I sat on the sidelines at Rae Rae's soccer practice without having a coughing fit or dragging an oxygen tank behind me. Even walking around aimlessly in Kroger with Robert was joyous. With every achievement, I just shook my head and praised God for bringing me through.

I went back to work full time in late March 2017, approximately five months after my transplant. My doctors and coordinators in Baltimore said that my quick return to work was out of the ordinary and even downright amazing. I shared my story with pre-transplant patients and followed up with all the churches, organizations, and individuals who had prayed for me. I believe that prayer works and that there is incredible power released from heaven when groups of people pray together. In my situation, there was nothing else anyone could do. I couldn't organize it, orchestrate it, or manage it. Only God could have made my transplant happen, and looking back, His hand was on my life every step of the way.

At every point in this journey—on the good days and the really horrible ones—I could always look back and see good things God had done. He was always faithful and always with me. He was always good and always in control, even when I had no idea what the next minute held. No matter what, I knew I was winning, and nothing could change that ...

... not even the most unexpected loss of them all.

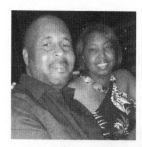
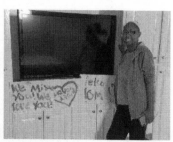

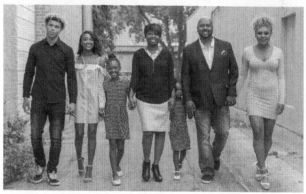

SEVENTEEN

... And Now This?

"MOM. IT'S LATE, AND WE'RE not at school." I looked at
my phone and noticed it was 9:34 a.m. Why was Raelyn
calling me from the house phone? Was it Saturday?

A week earlier, my friends Tamara, Jessica, and I had
decided we would spend the night at Tamara's house
after the Tuesday night Beyoncé concert we had tickets
for. We'd make a girls' night out of it and celebrate
Jessica's birthday with brunch and a trip to the spa on
Wednesday before heading home. I informed Robert of
our plan. He was onboard and happy that I was getting
out for some fun with my girlfriends. It had been nearly
two years since my transplant, and he and I had
continued to live life fully. The Tuesday of the concert
came, and I had a 7:00 a.m. meeting scheduled at work,
so I needed to leave Denton by 6:00 a.m. to get there
on time. I woke up and got dressed, then walked over
to Rob's side of the bed to tell him I was heading out.
"Hey, I'm gone. The girls' clothes are on the ironing

board. Don't forget that I'm seeing Bey tonight, so I'll see you Wednesday evening. I love you and will give you a buzz when I get to work." I bent down and gave Robert a kiss and a hug.

"Aight. Have fun. I'll get up in a bit. Love you too," he replied.

Our day was typical. We talked throughout the day. He called me while he was doing his daily Kroger run. He had a hankering for roast and wanted my opinion on if he should cook one or two. I reminded him I didn't care what he cooked because I would be with Beyoncé for dinner. He had closed on his first house that day and had texted me pictures of him and his clients together at closing. Late that afternoon, he had met with another client who was having an inspection completed and then had scooped the girls up from the house to take them to STEM night at their school. I called him when I left work headed to Tamara's and again when we were on our way to the concert. Then I texted him throughout the concert.

At the concert, I thought about how fabulous it was to be out with my girlfriends with no complaints from my husband. Still, I found myself wishing he was there. We were the best companions and just had a vibe that flowed. We had perfected our routine, and it felt strange to break from it. The concert ended around midnight, and when we finally made it to the car, I called Robert. I told him all about the concert and how we were sitting in awful traffic. Robert was glad I had had a good time and told me about the evening he'd spent with the girls. He told me he would call me back, which

I knew typically just meant "goodbye." I said, "I love you."

He said, "I love you too."

We hung up.

At 9:34 a.m., Raelyn called.

"So, wake Daddy up," I instructed her. I could hear her walking into our bedroom and calling out to Robert. I questioned her waking strategy. "Are you shaking him? Are you talking loud? Are y'all playing a joke?" I told her I'd call her right back and called Robert's phone. He would never sleep through his cell phone ringing, but there was no answer. I called Rae back, and she kept telling me that Daddy was not waking up. I could hear our nephew, Jamaras, in the background. I told Rae to put him on the phone.

"Jamaras, the girls are super late for school. Go wake Robert up."

I could hear him walk into our room and call out to Robert. "Sir. Sir. Uncle Robert. Wow, he's really sleeping."

I yelled through the phone, "Is he not responding? What's going on!?"

Jamaras answered, "No."

"Call 911 right now!" I yelled.

I ran into Tamara's living room and told her that we had to get to Denton. Robert wasn't responding, and I didn't know what was happening. I grabbed my things and called Jamaras back. I handed the phone off to Tamara as I finished getting dressed. She said she could hear them doing CPR. We rushed out of the door. I called my in-laws and told them Robert wasn't

142

responding and they needed to get to my house immediately. I then tried to call my neighbors but couldn't remember what the contacts icon on my phone looked like. I was trembling and cumbersome. I couldn't believe what could be happening. I called Jamaras back.

"Mimi ... he's gone."

"What do you mean, he's gone?"

"Mimi, he passed ... he's gone."

I screamed from the bottom of my soul, tears soaking my face. I was shaking and crying and repeating "NO" over and over in disbelief and shock. I called my pastor, Robert's childhood friends, my mom, Robert and Telia's mom, and Jasmine. Each conversation was surreal: "Hey ... Robert's gone ... Yes ... We don't know ... Rae found him unresponsive ... He passed."

When Rae first called me, the possibility that Robert could be dead was not even a thought. After all we had been through, God would take him away on a random Tuesday night? This could not be real. He was just fine. He had gotten a clean bill of health just three weeks before. We had plans. He had just closed his first real estate deal. I was healthy. The kids were doing well in school. We were living our best life. I just talked to him last night. *What the hell?*

Tamara and I arrived at our house in Denton to a multitude of cars and a swelling crowd of long-faced people. Police cars and cars of family lined the streets around our home. Neighbors stood on their porches and on the sidewalk across from our house. I remember how eerily quiet it was when I exited the car even though there were dozens of people outside. I walked into the house and was met by a detective who told me he was sorry for my loss and then proceeded to ask me questions. They wouldn't let me in the room, and honestly, I didn't want to see my Love like that. I looked for Rae and Londy and found them on the couch soaking in tears. All I could do was hug their heads and say I was sorry. I started hearing people come in, wailing. I remember people touching my shoulders affectionately and reminding me to eat and take my meds. As I ate some of the leftover roast Robert had made the night before, all I could think about was that my best friend had died and how everything was going to fall on my shoulders. *Now, I gotta raise these kids by my damn self! The mortgage. His truck. Did I just take my last vacation? Was he in pain? Did he know? I have to stay healthy for real now. Oh, God! This is crazy!*

I told my pastor how I knew all the things that are supposed to be true—the "right" things people say—during a situation like this. God makes no mistakes. God is good. God is my Provider and Supplier and Comforter. Blessed are those who mourn, for they shall be comforted. God is the great I AM. But, in that moment, I didn't see the benefit of Robert dying. *What good could come of this? What good could come of the fact that our five year old will live the rest of her life without her Daddy … that Raelyn had to be the one to discover him and will have those images in her head the rest of her life … that he won't be here to see Jasmine walk across the stage at her college graduation in three months … that he won't be here for Robert Jr.'s or Telia's*

144

graduations ... that all our plans had been interrupted and denied in an instant. What is the benefit?

It seemed ironic that I was not the first to go. We often joked about me going first, what kind of funeral I wanted, and how he was going to be a rich man in every way. We had just assumed that I would go first, not anytime soon, but first. Now, we're stuck trying to figure out how to cope with the loss of him.

I began reciting Jeremiah 29:11 over and over: "'For I know the plans I have for you,' declares the LORD, 'plans to prosper you and not to harm you, plans to give you hope and a future.'" I kept reminding myself that there is a plan. It's not anything like the plan we had in mind, but it is a plan none the less. We weren't going to be in the poor house. We would get through this and carry on *His* plan no matter what.

We all had our moments of extreme grief over the week and a half before Robert's homegoing celebration. I think I cried in my car in parking lots all over the Dallas-Fort Worth Metroplex. I stayed busy planning his service, going through old pictures and videos, and crying. It was difficult to comfort and console all the kids, our family, our friends, and myself at the same time, especially when the one who usually comforted me was not available ... and never would be. I thought about Jesus' words in John 16:33: "These things I have spoken unto you, that in me ye might have peace. In the world ye shall have tribulation: but be of good cheer; I have overcome the world" (King James Version).

To me, this verse meant that Jesus understood what I was going through. He had experienced grief and unfathomable pain. He knew what it was like to cry out to God, His tears like drops of blood. And still, He had overcome. I would overcome as well. It would be alright. Hard and painful, but eventually alright. I met with friends who were widows and sought out counseling for all of us. Our family and friends descended upon us. They loved and fed us. Our church family embraced us. The elementary school where Rae and Londy attend called immediately and supported us. My director, co-workers, and hospital administrators supported me through it all.

There were over six hundred people in attendance at Robert's service. It was a true testament of his life of fun, giving, and love. Still, it was hard knowing that this was real, that he was really gone. During the days leading up to the celebration, I received numerous texts, calls, and personal recounts from people I knew and didn't really know. They shared stories of how Robert had helped them at some point in their lives. He was doing a lot of good in the world, and like his friend Alex said, "Robert was rarely on time, but he was in our lives at the right time."

Personally, I am so grateful that he was my husband and advocate throughout my sickness. Without question, I would not be alive today if it had not been for him.

AS I SAW IT

All the time I think about what our life would be like had Lia not made it. *How would the girls be? How would I recover? How would I manage?* It's just crazy how everything came together and just flowed. If we had gone left instead of right, things would have been completely different.

—Robert Young (one week before he passed)

I've realized that I shouldn't try to understand why Robert passed. It didn't and still doesn't make sense. It may never. Yet, in my head and heart, I've decided that Robert was sent for a purpose. That purpose was different to everyone he knew, loved, and interacted with. His purpose in my life was to save it, and he had done just that. Believing this comforted me. Robert's job was done.

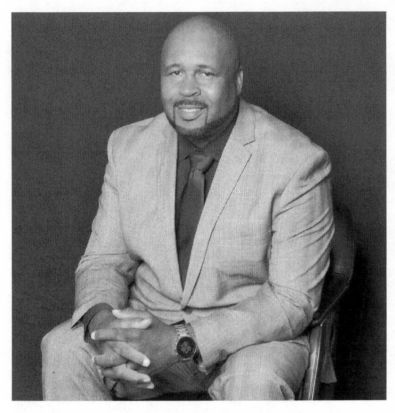

I have fought the good fight, I have finished the race,

I have kept the faith.

2 Timothy 4:7

Epilogue

SINCE ROBERT'S PASSING, life has been different, very different. I realize that there are single parents who run their households every day with amazing proficiency, but this is new to me. This new normal is hard, strange, and yet, sometimes and in some ways, carries unexpected splashes of beauty. I feel that Robert's absence has forced me to be better in all areas of my life. A better mother. More organized. A better steward of finances and planning for the future. Even a chef in my own right. In this new normal, I can breathe, participate in my kids' activities, and teach them how to navigate puberty and young adulthood. In this new normal, I climb into bed alone every night; remember Robert looking like Bluto as he dyed his beard at the bathroom sink; consider whether I now check the "single," "married," or "widowed" box on forms; and laugh by myself at our inside jokes. In this new normal, I also get to watch Jasmine cross the stage at her college graduation and read the letter of acceptance for Raelyn into private school. I get to say, "Rob, we did it."

I miss Robert immensely, and our family and community do as well. His absence affects each of our daily routines. It has been emotionally draining for me to "be strong," grieve, and wipe everybody else's tears and my own at the same time. I can't call Robert on the way to work or throughout the day. I can't ask him important questions as they cross my mind or let him know how my treatments went. I must make decisions I never thought I'd make alone. I have to coordinate getting the kids home from school, what we're going to eat, and when and where to get groceries. Y'all, I even have to pump my own gas and clean my car! Most importantly, I don't get to hug, kiss, laugh, or dream with him anymore.

Initially, I kept saying how crazy Robert's passing was. (And it is crazy—we're still a little in shock and disbelief.) I tried hard to see the benefit of losing my best friend and lifesaver. But I think I'm done searching for something I may never find. Instead, I'm finding comfort in the love and support of our friends, family, and community. And I'm choosing to do what I did at other times when the journey didn't make sense—I'm remembering what God did before and trusting Him for what I can't see yet.

I felt at peace after the celebration service and determined that something really good—beyond anything I can ask for or imagine—was coming for my "boo" to be gone. When I was sick, Robert and I prayed that I would live to see my children's children's children. However, we never prayed for Robert. I believe that part of Robert's purpose in life was to save mine so that the answer to our prayers could manifest, and I could live to know my great-grandchildren, even if he isn't here to witness it.

In this new normal, I will continue to trust God because He is God. He is Love. He is Healer. And He is working for my good. Always.

This is my new normal, and no matter what, I *still* win.

Frequently Asked Questions

What is scleroderma?
Scleroderma is a chronic auto immune disease in which the body attacks its own connective tissue. Connective tissue holds the organs together and is also found in joints. The word *scleroderma* means "hard skin," and the most visible manifestation of the disease is hard, tight skin. In some cases, scleroderma can affect internal organs rather than (or in addition to) the skin. It is unknown how you get this rare disease, and it usually affects women more than men. Its onset is usually between the ages of 25–55. There is no cure, but the symptoms can be managed. The degree to which it affects a person varies from person to person. Some patients are on no medications while others are wheelchair bound due to immobility because of their tightening skin. Scleroderma is not cancer. It is also not contagious, malignant, or infectious.

How (and why) did you research being double listed?
All my life, I have been the type to seek all possible information before making a decision. When National Jewish Hospital in Denver informed me that I would probably need a lung transplant in my lifetime, I began reading everything available. I remember one of the articles describing the process for getting listed mentioned "dual listing." There are special requirements to meet and agreements to make in order to be dual listed. As the months went by with no

transplant, becoming dual listed was a necessity and priority to me.

Why is it always worth it to get a second (and third or fourth) opinion?

Simply put, your life depends on it. It is the PRACTICE of medicine. New innovations, methods, and research are becoming available every day. One physician or facility may perform a procedure better or more efficiently than another. In my scenario, I wanted the best and was willing to do whatever was necessary to be seen by the best. You have to get a second opinion, so you can make an informed decision about your health and your life. Had I not sought out a second opinion when my "pneumonia" came back a third time, I could have easily digressed into a state where I was too sick to have options. It is my opinion that you need to act quickly, get a second opinion, and never stop seeking help until your issue is resolved.

Why should a patient do his or her own research and ask questions? Isn't the doctor always right?

I cannot impress upon you enough how important it is to do your research, be your own advocate, and have someone who loves you and knows your wishes be your advocate. Even though I am in the healthcare field, I was unfamiliar with the transplant world. I had to do a significant amount of research and inquiry on my own. My home team did not provide information for me about new innovations and treatments. I get it. There is a bottom line to maintain, and one team doesn't want to promote another facility. That would be like someone who works for Whataburger saying, "You know, our chicken sandwich is good, but you should go across the street to Chick– fil-A for a real chicken sandwich." That's just not done. I shared the information I had learned with Robert, Tamara, and my mom, asked my providers lots of questions, and followed up with the transplant team on their stated plan of care and other things they said they were going to do. Yes, I was THAT patient. I joined support groups, talked with current and former patients, and was very transparent on social media about what I was going through. I wanted to know everything about my condition and the physicians managing my care. It was a fulltime job managing my health, but it allowed me to make informed decisions and limited the number of surprises I encountered.

Why did you have to go through so much just to get on the transplant list?
Every transplant center is trying to provide excellent patient care, help people get well, and get good results, which is determined by longer mortality for patients. The difficult reality is that for many transplants to happen, a donor must die. Therefore, donated organs are a precious and scarce commodity, and transplant centers try to choose recipients with the best possible chance of being saved, ensuring the maximum impact of every donated organ. Additionally, transplant centers are monitored by the Center for Medicare and Medicaid (CMS). For centers to qualify for reimbursement by the

CMS, they must meet certain criteria, among which are patient survival rates. This puts a lot of pressure on centers not to transplant many high-risk patients. Consequently, the transplant centers assess each candidate from various angles—financial, physical, social, and spiritual—and choose those they determine have the best chance of survival and long-term mortality.

What information did you learn on your journey that was most helpful?

The most helpful information was the information I learned by attending scleroderma support group meetings in my local area and through the Facebook lung transplant support group. As a newly diagnosed scleroderma patient, I was scared and had a lot of questions. The group meetings confirmed that I was not alone and helped answer my questions. The lung transplant group had the same effect. It was good to know that others had the same questions and concerns I had. It was also encouraging to see survivors who had reached their 10-, 15-, and 20-year "lung-aversaries."

Could the scleroderma come back?

This is an excellent question. One for which I really don't have a clear answer. My scleroderma manifested only in my lungs, as far as we know. Now that I have new lungs, one would think that I have been cured from the disease. However, scleroderma is a chronic disease. Even though I have not had any of the symptoms of scleroderma that I had prior to the transplant, I assume there is a chance that it could pop its head up somewhere else. I am on immunosuppressants to prevent organ rejection and essentially suppress my immune system. I remain prayerful and hopeful that I will live to see the promises God has over my life with no issues from scleroderma.

Is the life expectancy post lung transplant still only five years? If so, why?

The lungs are more susceptible to infection and damage than any other organ. Every time I breathe, I am exposing my lungs to potential harm. My lungs are not protected like the heart, kidney, or liver. According to the National Institutes of Health (NIH), 78% of patients survive the first year, 63% of patients survive three years, and 51% survive five years after a lung transplant.[1] I try not to think about the stats for life expectancy and instead think of how blessed I am that my life has been extended. I think of how bad my health was in 2016 and how good it is now. I make a concerted effort to live life to the fullest and take advantage of all oppor-tunities. Robert's unexpected passing reinforced the fact that tomorrow is not promised. It has been challenging trying to balance protecting my health and taking advantage of all opportunities.

---

[1] "Pulmonary Fibrosis Lung Transplant." *Pulmonary Fibrosis News*, 15 Nov. 2016, pulmonaryfibrosisnews.com/pulmonary-fibrosis-lung-transplant.

So how are you now, healthwise?

I visited my doctor in Baltimore in March 2018. They notified me in April that they saw donor specific antibodies (DSA's). These are antibodies that come from the donor organ and can potentially cause rejection of the organ. The appearance of these is anticipated, and the amount found was not critical. In response to this finding, I had a port placed in my chest and started photopharesis treatments in July. Photopharesis is a process where they remove blood via my port, spin it, add a medication, flash the blood with UV light, and return it back to me. It doesn't hurt, and there are basically no after effects. I do have to wear sunscreen and sunglasses to protect my skin and eyes. Lab results in early 2019 indicated that I should be able to stop photopheresis. In February 2019, I visited my doctor in Baltimore, and he confirmed what the lab results suggested, officially taking me off photopheresis. Otherwise, I've been great. No rejection, infection, or issues since the transplant.

What advice would you give to others who are awaiting a transplant or going through a medical crisis?

1. Pray without ceasing. Have others pray for and with you.

2. Learn to let go. This was hard for me, but when I became really sick, I quickly realized that God was in control. There was absolutely nothing that I could do to fix my situation. I had to focus on enjoying the time I had, being a compliant patient, and trusting God to take

care of everything. I accepted that I could die but realized that regardless of the outcome, I would be victorious.

3.   Start fundraising and saving your money immediately. Costs will arise that insurance will not cover. You will need cash, and possibly a lot of it. If you can't physically fundraise, designate someone who loves you to be your chief fundraiser.

4.   Get familiar with your insurance benefits and coverage. Know your benefits coordinator at your place of employment, if applicable.

5.   You need to have serious, uncomfortable conversations with your spouse, children, parents, and close friends about your end-of-life wishes. These desires need to be made known, put on paper, documented, and filed. You need a living will which is a document that gives your physicians and treatment team instructions on what treatments you do and do not want should you be incapacitated. You need a durable medical power of attorney. This document tells the world who makes medical decisions for you. The designee will be the one who gets all of the information from physicians, makes the decisions on your behalf, and fills in the gaps where your living will is unclear. Finally, get a will. Everybody needs a will regardless of your tax bracket. Don't let your lack of preparation leave your family at odds with each other. I am not an attorney, and the laws are different between states. Know the laws in your state.

How did you explain your condition to your kids?
Robert and I were very honest and open about my condition with our children. We did our best to talk to them on their level. When we got back from Denver, we told them that I had scleroderma and what it was. We informed them that I would have to perform several tests and possibly get a double lung transplant. When I became active on the transplant list, we told them that my lungs were damaged, and I needed new ones. We told them that we wouldn't know when the lungs would be ready, but someone had to pass and give them to Mommy. When I was hospitalized prior to the transplant, I requested that my friends and co-workers who are Childlife Specialists talk to the kids about my illness and the possibility of me dying.

How do I get in contact with your doctor in Baltimore?
Currently (at the time this book was published), Dr. Aldo Iacono practices at the University of Maryland Medical Center at 16 S. Eutaw Street in Baltimore, Maryland. The phone number to the lung transplant department is 410-328-2864.

What did people say to you when you were sick that was NOT helpful?
There was a handful of people who probably meant well but should have just kept quiet. When I announced that I needed a double lung transplant, these people approached me and/or messaged me to say they felt so sorry for me and that my situation was "so horrible." Now, I was not in denial about my situation. I knew it

was bad, and I had a lot of questions. My future was uncertain. The last thing I wanted to hear was someone telling me how bad off I was. I was not having a pity party and didn't want anyone hosting one for me.

What did they say or do that WAS helpful?
As mentioned in the book, hundreds (if not thousands!) of people were praying for me. People sent me Bible verses and prayers around the clock when I was sick. These words of encouragement always seemed to appear in my inbox at the right time. Post-transplant, as I was discussing all I needed and wanted to do, my friend and co-worker Sherry commented that Rome was not built in a day. That simple comment helped me put things in perspective and be patient about regaining everything I had missed while waiting for my transplant.

What did people say to you when Robert passed that was NOT helpful?
When Robert passed, we were all in shock. Most people hugged me, cried, and shook their heads in disbelief. There were no words. However, someone told me that I was "unlucky." This was not something I wanted to hear, nor was it something I chose to believe.

What did they say or do when Robert passed that WAS helpful?
I met with several friends who had lost their husbands unexpectedly. Each of them encouraged me to do what felt right for me at the time. There were no rules, requirements, or expectations for how I should deal

with the loss of Robert. I appreciated hearing this over and over. It gave me permission to just be me and let my emotions do what they needed to do. I cried when I felt the need. I talked to him when I needed to. I didn't do anything I didn't want to do. And, I took time to myself just to think and to process everything that had happened.

What language, books, or services do you recommend for children who have experienced the death of a parent?

I acquired counseling for the kids and myself soon after Robert's passing. We attended group grief counseling meetings called Safe Haven that the kids enjoyed. My Childlife Specialist friends came again to talk with the kids the weekend after Robert's passing. They brought several books and resources, which I have listed at the end of the FAQs. It was difficult to find a therapist in our area for Londyn because of her age, but after two months of researching, we found a play therapist who specializes in grief. We are currently in the thick of all this as I finalize the editing of this story. Every day presents the opportunity to discover what stage of grieving each family member is in and how to cope with grief and each other. It remains to be seen if any of my efforts and counseling have been beneficial, but, as always, I remain hopeful.

Book List

These books have helped my daughters and me as we process and grieve Robert's passing:

How I Feel: A Coloring Book For Grieving Children. By Alan D. Wolfelt, Ph.D.

What Will I Tell the Children: Helping Your Children Cope with Death. Nebraska Medicine.

Remember... A Child Remembers: A Write-in Memory Book for Grieving Children. By Enid Samuel-Traisman, M.S.W. (This was a journal with questions that prompt the child to write the memories she has of the deceased loved one.)

Love Never Stops: A Memory Book for Children. By Emilio Parga, M.A. (This is another journal/scrapbook with prompts for pictures and memories.)

Medical Terms Glossary

Advanced lung disease team: a group of healthcare providers that specializes in treating diseases of the lung such as chronic obstructive pulmonary disease (COPD), emphysema, asthma, and interstitial lung disease.

Albuterol: a medication, usually delivered through an inhaler or nebulizer, that relaxes the muscles in the airways and increases air flow to the lungs.

Ambulatory: related to walking; able to walk and move about independently.

Anesthesia: medications intended to numb sensation to part or all of the body.

Anesthesiologist: a medical doctor who specializes in caring for patients and their pain relief/anesthesia needs before, during, and after surgery.

Antibodies: the major component of the immune system; proteins that are found in the blood whose sole purpose is to attack foreign invaders (antigens) in the body; antibodies are produced naturally and can also be obtained through pregnancy and blood product transfusions. In organ transplantation, antibody classes that are a high percentage in the potential recipient need to be matched between the donor and recipient in order to prevent chronic rejection of the transplanted organ.

Antibiotic: type of medication used in the treatment and prevention of bacterial infections.

Antigens: a toxin or other foreign substance that induces an immune response in the body, especially the production of antibodies; examples are bacteria, fungi, or viruses.

AP (anterior – posterior) image: an x-ray image taken from front to back.

Arthritis: a general term for joint pain or joint disease.

Aspirate: to breathe or swallow something foreign into the lungs.

BiPAP machine: bilevel positive airway pressure; a form of ventilation delivered by a tight-fitting mask; a BiPap machine helps push air into the lungs. The machine provides pressurized air into the airways, which opens the lungs.

Breathing Treatments: medication delivered via a nebulizer to help a patient breathe.

Bronchoscopy: a procedure that looks inside the patient's airway and lungs. It involves inserting a scope tube with a camera at the end through the nose or mouth, down the throat, into the trachea (windpipe), and to the lungs.

Caesarian section (C-section): a surgical childbirth procedure in which the baby is removed from the mother's uterus.

Cardiothoracic surgeon: a medical doctor who specializes in the surgical treatment of internal organs, specifically the lungs and heart.

Catheter: thin tube placed in the body for medical purposes.

Chemotherapy: a type of cancer treatment in which one or more anti-cancer drugs are administered to the patient.

Chest tube: a flexible plastic tube that is inserted through the chest wall to drain blood or fluid or to relieve air.

Chronic: persisting for a long time or constantly recurring.

CPAP machine: continuous positive airway pressure; a form of ventilation delivered by a tight-fitting mask. A CPAP machine sends a constant flow of airway pressure to the throat to ensure that the airway stays open.

Crepitus: the grating, crackling, or popping sounds and sensations caused by air in body tissue.

CT scan (computerized tomography): a medical imaging scan that combines a series of x-ray images taken from different angles to produce cross-sectional images of a part of the body. It provides more detailed images than a simple x-ray.

Cytoxan: a drug used to treat certain types of cancer by decreasing the response of the patient's immune system to various diseases.

Dermatologist: a medical doctor who specializes in the treatment of skin issues and diseases.

Dietician: a medical professional who specializes in using food and nutrition to promote health and manage disease.

Dual listed: when one patient is on the transplant list at two different hospitals, transplant centers, or medical networks.

ECMO (extracorporeal membrane oxygenation): a form of respiratory life support. The ECMO machine pumps and oxygenates a patient's blood outside the body in the machine, allowing the heart and lungs to rest.

Emergency Medical Technician (EMT): a healthcare provider who provides care in an ambulance.

Epidural: a process in which anesthesia medication is injected near the spinal cord in order to block the nerves and deaden sensation.

Esophagus: the muscular tube connecting the throat to the stomach.

Extubate: to remove the long tube that is connected to a ventilator and runs from the ventilator, through the mouth, down the throat, and into the lungs.

Flurries: (as in a chest x-ray): unknown objects seen on an x-ray; looks like snow flurries or dandelions.

Gastrointestinal reflux disease (GERD): occurs when stomach acid frequently flows back into the esophagus; also called acid reflux.

Gynecologist: medical doctor who specializes in the health of the female reproductive system and breasts.

Hemorrhaging: bleeding in profuse amounts.

Hydrocodone 10mg: prescriptive drug used for treating severe pain.

Hyperglycemia: high blood sugar.

IVC (inferior vena cava) filter: a type of vascular filter that is implanted to prevent blood clots.

ICU: Intensive Care Unit of a hospital.

Immune system: the body's defense against infectious organisms; it is made up of a network of cells, tissues, and organs that work together to protect the body.

Immunologist: a medical doctor who specializes in managing problems related to the immune system, such as allergies and autoimmune diseases.

Immunosuppressive drugs: medications that lower the body's ability to fight foreign organisms or organs that may appear foreign.

Infectious disease doctors: medical doctors who specialize in the diagnosis, control, and treatment of infections.

Internal medicine: medical specialty dealing with the prevention, diagnosis, and treatment of adult diseases.

Intubation: the placement of a flexible plastic tube into the trachea (windpipe) to maintain an open airway.

IV (intravenous): the insertion of a tube into a vein.

Labor and Delivery: the department at hospitals and medical centers that specialize in the birthing process.

Lasix: a diuretic (water pill) that helps your body get rid of excess fluid.

LAT image: x-ray image taken laterally (from side to side).

LOVENOX: a medicine used to prevent and treat harmful blood clots.

Lungs: the primary organs of the respiratory system; humans have two lungs, which are located near the backbone on either side of the heart.

Lung Allocation Score (LAS): this score is used to prioritize lung transplant waiting list candidates based on a combination of waitlist urgency, current medical condition, and likelihood of post-transplant survival.

Lung biopsy: a procedure in which samples of lung tissue are removed (with a special biopsy needle or during surgery) to determine if lung disease or cancer is present.

Lung (VQ) scan: an imaging test that uses a ventilation (V) scan to measure air flow in the lungs and a perfusion (Q) scan to see where blood flows in the lungs.

Lupus: an autoimmune disease, which happens when the immune system attacks its own tissue, causing inflammation, swelling, pain, and damage.

Magnetic Resonance Imaging (MRI): a form of medical imaging that uses strong magnetic fields to produce images of internal organs.

Morphine: a prescription drug used to treat moderate to severe pain.

Lactation Nurse: a registered nurse who helps train and meet the needs of breastfeeding mothers.

Nasal cannula: a device used to deliver supplemental oxygen to patients who need respiratory help; it consists of a lightweight tube that attaches to an oxygen tank on one end and divides on the other into two prongs, which are placed in the patient's nostrils.

Neonatal Intensive Care Unit (NICU): an intensive care unit specializing in the care of ill or premature newborns.

Non-specific interstitial pneumonia (NSIP): a rare disorder that affects the tissue that surrounds and separates the tiny air sacs of the lungs. These air sacs, called the alveoli, are where the exchange of oxygen and carbon dioxide takes place between the lungs and the bloodstream.

Nurse Practitioner: a nurse who is qualified to treat certain medical conditions without the direct supervision of a doctor.

Obstetrician (OB): a medical doctor who specializes in the care and treatment of pregnant women and women in childbirth.

Occupational Therapist (OT): a therapist who helps patients regain and rehabilitate the skills and functions required in daily life.

Open lung biopsy: an invasive procedure requiring general anesthesia, in which the chest is cut open in order to remove a large lung tissue sample.

Oxygen converter: a machine that takes air from the environment and converts it into oxygen. It delivers the oxygen to the patient via tubing and a nasal cannula.

Oxygen saturation (O2 sats): refers to the extent to which the blood is saturated with oxygen. Normal levels for humans are between 95—100%. Percentages below 90% are considered low and require supplemental oxygen.

PEG (Percutaneous endoscopic gastrostomy) tube: a tube that is passed into a patient's stomach through the abdominal wall to provide a means of feeding when oral intake is not adequate or appropriate.

Physical Therapist (PT): a therapist who helps patients regain or rehabilitate physical movements through activity and exercise or who treats disease and injury through physical methods.

Physician's Fellow: a medical doctor who recently completed his or her residency and is in a one-year period of specialized training called a Fellowship.

PH probe: a 24-hour test that uses a thin probe or tube placed in the esophagus or food pipe that connects the mouth to the stomach to help diagnose and treat acid reflux.

PICC line (peripherally inserted central catheter): a thin, soft, long catheter (tube) that is inserted into a vein in the arm, leg, or neck. The PICC line is used for long-term intravenous (IV) antibiotics, nutrition or medications, and for blood draws.

Pitting enema: when a person places a finger on his or her leg, removes it, and the imprint stays.

Plasmapheresis: a procedure in which blood plasma is removed, treated, and returned to the body.

Pneumonia: an infection of the lungs in which they are inflamed and the air sacs are often filled with fluid or pus; can cause severe cough, fever, chills, and difficulty breathing.

Pneumothorax: a collapsed lung.

Post-op: after operation. For example, a "post-op" room is where a patient is brought immediately after a medical procedure, such as a surgery.

Prednisone: an anti-inflammatory steroid medication used to treat a variety of conditions.

Psychologist: a professional with a degree in psychology who studies the mental state, human behavior, and human emotions and aids patients in their mental health and well-being.

Pulmonary embolism: artery blockage between the heart and lungs.

Pulmonary fibrosis: scarring in the lungs.

Pulmonary hypertension: a serious medical condition that results when the arteries carrying blood to the lungs are constricted and the blood flow is disrupted.

Pulmonologist: a medical doctor who specializes in respiratory (lung/breathing-related) diseases.

Pulse oximeter: a method for monitoring a patient's oxygen saturation.

Raynaud's: a condition marked by numbness of finger tips in response to cold temperatures.

Resident: a medical doctor who holds a medical degree and is completing a period of specialized training called a "residency."

Respiratory system: the body system that consists of organs and structures related to breathing (inhaling and exhaling).

Respiratory Therapist (RT): a therapist who assesses and treats patients with acute and/or chronic dysfunction of the cardiopulmonary (heart and respiratory) systems.

Rheumatologist: a medical doctor who specializes in the diagnosis and treatment of musculoskeletal and autoimmune diseases.

Sarcoidosis: (SAR-COY-DOE-SIS) an inflammatory disease characterized by the formation of granulomas—tiny clumps of inflammatory cells—in one or more organs of the body. When the immune system goes into overdrive and too many of these clumps form, they can interfere with an organ's structure and function. When left unchecked, chronic inflammation can lead to fibrosis, which is the permanent scarring of organ tissue. This disorder affects the lungs in approximately 90% of cases, but it can affect almost any organ in the body.

Scleroderma: (also called "systemic sclerosis") a chronic connective tissue autoimmune disease.

Six-minute walk test: an exercise test that measures the distance walked over a span of six minutes.

Skin contractures: a deformity resulting from the tightening of skin.

Speech Therapist: a therapist trained to help patients develop or recover a full range of speech sounds and speech.

Steroids (Corticosteroids): cortisone-like medicines; used to provide relief for inflamed areas of the body. They lessen swelling, redness, itching, and allergic reactions.

Spirometry: (spy-ROM-uh-tree) a common office test used to assess how well the lungs work by measuring how much air the patient inhales, how much she exhales, and how quickly she exhales.

Swallow test (barium swallow test): used to diagnose disorders that make swallowing difficult or affect the esophagus, stomach, and the first part of the small intestine. The barium swallow test is a special kind of x-ray test that allows the doctor to view the back of the patient's mouth, throat, and esophagus.

Tacrolimus: an immunosuppressant medication prescribed to prevent organ transplantation rejection.

Trachea: commonly referred to as the "windpipe," a tube about four inches in length that allows the passages of air into the lungs.

Tracheal deviation: a shift of the trachea to the left or right of its normal position.

Transplantation: (of organs) replacing organs with the organs from another person; some organs are from living donors and some are not.

United Network for Organ Sharing (UNOS): the private, non-profit organization that manages the nation's organ transplant system.

Urinary catheter: (often called a "Foley catheter") a small tube inserted into the urethra to drain the bladder.

VATS (Video Assisted Thoracoscopic Surgery): a minimally invasive surgical technique used to diagnose and treat problems in the chest.

Ventilator: an appliance that provides artificial respiration.

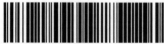

36482280R00107

Made in the USA
San Bernardino, CA
21 May 2019